The Educated Heart

Professional Boundaries for Massage Therapists, Bodyworkers, and Movement Teachers

SECOND EDITION

The Educated Heart

Professional Boundaries for Massage Therapists, Bodyworkers, and Movement Teachers

SECOND EDITION

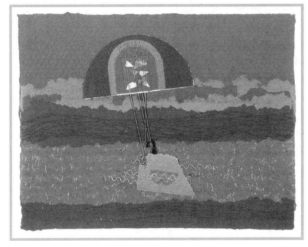

Nina McIntosh

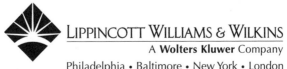

LWW In Touch Series

LIPPINCOTT WILLIAMS & WILKINS
A **Wolters Kluwer** Company

Philadelphia • Baltimore • New York • London
Buenos Aires • Hong Kong • Sydney • Tokyo

Senior Acquisitions Editor: Pete Darcy	*Cartoon Illustrations:* Mari Gayatri Stein
Development Editor: David Payne	*Cover Illustration:* Dolph Smith
Senior Marketing Manager: Christen D. Murphy	*Composition:* Lippincott Williams & Williams
Project Editor: Bill Cady	Desktop Composition
Designer: Risa Clow	*Printer:* Quebecor

Trademarks and Service Marks
- *Feldenkrais®* is a registered service mark of The FELDENKRAIS GUILD.®
- The word Rolfing® is a registered service mark of the Rolf Institute® of Structural Integration.
- *Trager®* is a registered service mark of the Trager Institute.
- Rubenfeld Synergy Method® is a registered service mark of the Rubenfeld Synergy Center and Ilana Rubenfeld.
- Rosen Method® is a registered service mark of the Rosen Institute.

Cover and chapter opening art: "Aslipah, Disguised As A River, Was Lowered Close To The Water By His Friends." Artist: Dolph Smith.

Handmade paper, original piece 18" x 24", Date: 1987. From the collection of and with the kind permission of Kathy Albers, Albers Gallery, Memphis, Tennessee.

This piece is part of the saga of the heroic journey of Aslipah, a paper airplane, and his struggle to prevail. Aslipah challenges the stereotype of being just "a slip of paper" and is embarked on a quest for the elusive meaning of life. Just as Aslipah is a symbol for everywoman/man's personal drama, his story is an apt metaphor for the journey of the manual therapies to reach a position of recognition and enlightenment.

Library of Congress Cataloging-in-Publication Data
McIntosh, Nina.
  The educated heart: professional boundaries for massage therapists, bodyworkers, and movement teachers / Nina McIntosh.—2nd ed.
    p. ; cm.
  Includes bibliographical references and index.
  ISBN-10: 0-7817-4886-0 (alk. paper) ISBN-13: 978-0-7817-4886-5
  1. Massage therapy—Practice. 2. Masseurs—Professional ethics. I. Title.
  [DNLM: 1. Massage. 2. Professional-Patient Relations. 3. Ethics, Professional. 4. Exercise Therapy. 5. Manipulation,
  Orthopedic. 6. Professional Practice—organization & administration. WB 537 M152e 2005]
RM722.M37 2005
615.8'22—dc22
                                                                                    2004021917

The publishers have made every effort to trace the copyright holders for borrowed material. If they have inadvertently overlooked any, they will be pleased to make the necessary arrangements at the first opportunity.

To purchase additional copies of this book, call our customer service department at **(800) 638-3030** or fax orders to **(301) 824-7390**. For other book services, including chapter reprints and large quantity sales, ask for the Special Sales Department. For all other calls originating outside of the United States, please call **(301)714-2324**.

Visit Lippincott Williams & Wilkins on the Internet: http://www.lww.com. Lippincott Williams & Wilkins customer service representatives are available from 8:30 am to 6:00 pm, EST, Monday through Friday, for telephone access.

08

4 5 6 7 8 9 10

Dedicated to the memory of my parents
who were always waiting
for me to get a real job.

ABOUT THE AUTHOR

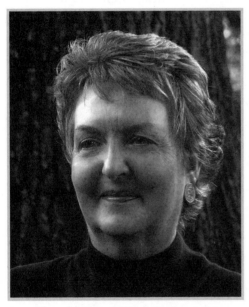

Photo by Elven Blalock Photography

For more than 25 years, Nina McIntosh's heart and interest have been with the world of the somatic therapies. Nina started her professional career in 1970 as a psychiatric social worker in Denver, Colorado, after receiving a Master of Social Work degree from Tulane University. She soon became intrigued by the therapeutic possibilities of the touch therapies; in 1978, she trained as a massage therapist at what is now the Boulder College of Massage Therapy. She became a certified Rolfer in 1981. In recent years, her interest in the psychological component of bodywork has led her to study Rosen Method bodywork at Rosen Method Center Southwest in Santa Fe, New Mexico.

Nina has long been a believer in the healing power of touch and has a broad knowledge of the manual therapies. Curiosity coupled with a desire to alleviate her own physical symptoms have led her to explore many different methods and techniques in depth. Aside from Rolfing and Rosen Method sessions, she has experienced the Trager Approach, craniosacral therapy, Aston Patterning, Healing Touch, Reiki, and most of the Asian modalities. She has taken extensive Feldenkrais movement classes and attended workshops in the Alexander technique and Lomi bodywork. Nina believes that each school and method has its own contribution to make and its own value for clients. Long a fan of massage therapy, she thinks that nothing is more valuable than the skill and artistry of a good massage.

Nina's training in professional boundaries began in her social work graduate program, where physical contact with clients was thought to be so potentially intrusive and unsettling that students were prohibited from touching clients. As she began to practice bodywork, she saw that manual therapists, who routinely cross that powerful physical boundary, could benefit from knowing more about how to create safe environments for their clients and themselves.

Nina opened up the discussion about boundaries and safety with the first edition of *The Educated Heart*, which became a standard text in many professional manual therapy programs. She also writes a column on professional boundaries, "The Heart of Bodywork," for *Massage & Bodywork* magazine.

Writing, teaching workshops, and doing consultations, Nina's wish is to give voice and validity to the experiences of somatic practitioners—to talk about what it is like on a day-to-day basis to be a massage therapist, bodyworker, or movement teacher. She wants to let manual therapists know that they are not alone and hopes to help both experienced practitioners and those just starting out create successful therapeutic relationships with their clients.

$\mathcal{F}$OREWORD

For years—decades, even—there have been no overview books covering the complexities of professional boundaries for those who are healers and helpers who communicate with the blessed body.

But now, with this new work by Nina McIntosh, brand-new massage students and advanced bodyworkers, massage therapists, and movement teachers alike, including practitioners of such disciplines as Feldenkrais, Alexander technique, Rosen Method bodywork, and others, will be likely to find this book not only useful and comprehensive but also recognize and feel "companioned" by the "inside skivvie" stories of the trade, told as only one from the inner circle of the profession can.

Too often, newly graduated, inexperienced, and temporarily stressed practitioners are left to find their own way and to make guesses about what is important or appropriate rather than having available a reference they can consult for reliable guidelines. This work puts so much of that to rest by giving practitioners reassuring vignettes, examples, and plentiful advice about what to do and, more importantly, what *not* to do. Here the author reveals critical information about cherishing the therapeutic relationship—that is, taking care of the details, boundaries, and nourishments of running a practice and serving one's clients. McIntosh generously shares solutions to many real-life conundrums, impasses, and other sensitive situations that face every professional.

Also, extending the natural wit and wisdom of the book are the illustrations. In the tradition of James Thurber and Nicole Hollander and other psychological cartoonists, the witty and charming cartoons of Mari Gayatri Stein grace this book. You will likely recognize yourself and others you know in these artful little gems.

When I first heard this book was in the works, I felt gladdened to know that the sharing of such important information would be available to all the deeply committed bodyworkers of the world and equally heartened to know that an insightful and sensitive woman would be writing it. Nina McIntosh has over 26 years of experience as either a bodyworker or a psychiatric social worker. She writes for caring bodyworkers who strive to protect both psyche and *soma*—that is, the body and soul of individuals who trustingly come to practitioners for help, strengthening, and a calming environs. This long-needed work is as much a companion for the journey as it is a book. And like a good companion, it is not only fascinating and lively, but it is also that most important of all qualities—it is *useful*.

June 1999
Clarissa Pinkola Estés, Ph.D.
Diplomate Jungian Analyst
Grievance Board Chair, State of Colorado

$\mathcal{P}$REFACE

The first edition of *The Educated Heart* was a pioneer in the field—the first book to focus solely on ethics and professional boundaries for the manual therapies. That edition was very well received by a profession that is realizing the importance of relationship skills in creating a safe and comfortable environment for both client and practitioner.

The first edition was also original in that it engaged readers with a conversational, nonjudgmental style, presented clear and easy-to-understand explanations of complex psychological dynamics, and brought dry concepts to life with real-life examples. It offered practical suggestions for everyday boundary situations and sound advice for both beginning and experienced practitioners. Lighthearted cartoon illustrations of common scenarios gave this sometimes anxiety-producing material a friendlier tone.

With this, the second edition, I have attempted to keep those popular and useful assets while reorganizing the material for greater clarity. Every chapter has been reorganized to make it easier to read and to teach and has been streamlined to avoid repetition of material. Furthermore, I have added some new features that I hope will both enhance readers' broader understanding of the dynamics of the client-practitioner relationship and give more specific tools for skillful interactions with clients.

Audience

This book is intended for all manual therapists or somatic practitioners, including massage therapists, bodyworkers, movement educators, practitioners of Asian methods, and practitioners who work primarily with energy fields. Additionally, it addresses the professional needs of manual therapists in all phases of their careers. For students, it offers the support and information needed to establish the solid professional boundaries that will be important for their success and well-being. For experienced practitioners, many of whom were never schooled in the complexities of client-practitioner relationships, it provides the chance to learn new ideas to make their practices more fulfilling or to reinforce their own good decisions. Also, it is written so that readers need no prior knowledge of psychological concepts to understand the dynamics presented.

Scope

The Educated Heart was never intended to be a comprehensive discussion of every aspect of our work. For instance, although it offers good basic information on setting up a business and on working with clients who have been physically or sexually abused, these areas are not covered in detail. Some subjects addressed in this book, such as working with clients who have been abused, are probably best learned through in-person workshops that offer experiential exercises and more complete instruction. Readers will need to seek out such workshops to receive proper training in these areas. Readers can also refer to the resources listed in "Appendix C: Related Readings" for more information on topics that are not covered in depth. Note, too, that this book is not intended as a substitute for learning your local and state ethics regulations, the requirements of your professional associations, or any relevant licensing requirements.

Although some of the finer points of working in a spa or a medical setting are not discussed here, the client-practitioner dynamics are the same in any environment. The focus of *The Educated Heart* on the vulnerability of our clients and the need to create safe, respectful relationships makes it a good resource for manual therapists practicing in any setting.

Overview

Below is an overview of the main concepts and tools presented in each chapter:

Chapter 1, "The Educated Heart: The Need for Professional Boundaries," covers why boundaries provide safety for both client and practitioner and why they are necessary in a professional relationship; it also presents seven major misconceptions about boundaries.

Chapter 2, "Protective Circles: Boundaries and the Professional Relationship," discusses the concept of boundaries as protective circles that show both client and practitioner what is appropriate inside the therapeutic relationship and what is not.

Chapter 3, "Framework: Nuts and Bolts of Boundaries," covers a wealth of nitty-gritty logistics and details of creating a professional environment, from advice about business cards to what to do if a regular client abruptly stops making appointments.

Chapter 4, "Client-Practitioner Dynamics: Boundaries and the Power Imbalance," discusses the concepts of transference and countertransference, including how transference creates a power difference that makes balance necessary and how countertransference can interfere with our compassion and objectivity.

Chapter 5, "Ethical Boundaries: From Theory to Practice," presents guidelines for making ethical decisions, including how to make judgment calls in ambiguous situations and discussions on such issues as informed consent, scope of practice, and confidentiality.

Chapter 6, "Boundaries and the Power of Words," is a new chapter that gives general guidelines for effective communication with clients and specific suggestions for what to say in common situations.

Chapter 7, "Sexual Boundaries: Protecting Our Clients," includes general concerns and specific help with maintaining appropriate sexual boundaries with clients, including clients who have been sexually abused or those who have a crush on their practitioners.

Chapter 8, "Sexual Boundaries: Protecting Ourselves," deals with such issues as protecting ourselves from clients who make inappropriate sexual remarks, knowing what to say or do when a client has an erection, and dealing with sexual predators within the profession.

Chapter 9, "Financial Boundaries: Getting Comfortable With Money," covers general attitudes about money that might get in the way of success; how to create financial policies that you are comfortable with; and the ins and outs of such issues as setting fees, charging for missed appointments, and giving refunds.

Chapter 10, "Dual Relationships and Boundaries: Wearing Many Hats," presents different kinds of dual relationships, including working with friends and family, converting clients into friends, and doing trades or bartering, and how to avoid or minimize common pitfalls.

Chapter 11, "Help With Boundaries: Support, Consultation, and Supervision," covers the need for getting outside help with client-practitioner dynamics as part of taking care of ourselves plus different kinds of outside help and the advantages of each.

New Content

Below is a list of new content features that have been added to this edition:

- A new chapter on communication with clients that covers how tone and attitude make a difference, cues for talking with clients during a session, and what to say in common problem situations.

- A new emphasis on protecting the professional rights of practitioners as well as taking care of clients, including the importance of the ability to set limits and suggestions for effectively doing so.

- More help with understanding the crucial concepts of transference and countertransference, including more case examples and new illustrations of how transference and countertransference might look in our relationships with clients.

- A clear summary of the elements necessary to a professional therapeutic relationship such as consistency and client-centered actions and words.

- A new illustration of what belongs in a therapeutic relationship and what does not.

- A more detailed discussion of outside help available to practitioners, including consultation, supervision, peer groups, and mentors. Case examples are given for how practitioners use these. Tips are also given for how to find a consultant or supervisor.

Key Features

The key learning features, many of which are new to this edition, are listed below:

- Case examples, highlighted in the text with a gray background, provide real-life examples of concepts and situations discussed in the text.
- Memorable quotes from the text are featured in the margins of each chapter.
- Key terms are boldfaced in the text and defined in the margins and in the glossary at the back of the book.
- Questions for Reflection help readers process and internalize the content presented in each chapter.
- Great illustrations by Mari Gayatri Stein are provided, including four new full-size cartoons and many new smaller gems.
- Lippincott Williams & Wilkins' Connection website offers teaching resources for instructors.

Final Thoughts

In writing this book, it was my wish to help this profession find the public recognition it deserves. Quite simply, I think the key to that recognition lies in the quality of our day-to-day interactions with clients. Before the first edition, I interviewed more than 50 experts in the profession about what makes a relationship healing. My conclusion could be summed up in a few words: treat yourself and your client with kindness and respect. For those of you who are interested in learning more about creating kind and respectful relationships, I hope this new edition will be a valuable resource and a useful friend.

$\mathcal{A}$CKNOWLEDGMENTS

I am so grateful to all the people who contributed to both editions of this book—to those who made sure the first edition got off the ground and to the friends and colleagues who shared valuable feedback and personal stories that added so much to the second edition. Many thanks also to those colleagues who expressed appreciation for the first edition and let me know how much it meant to them.

The artist, Mari Gayatri Stein, has been a constant delight to work with on both editions. Her amazing and quirky illustrations make manual therapists smile with recognition. The book wouldn't be nearly as interesting, and I wouldn't have had as much fun writing it without Mari and her lively feathered and furry friends.

The first edition never would have happened without the inspiration and support of Nan Narboe. In the early 1980s, she planted the seed for it in a talk she gave to the Rolf Institute. When I started writing in earnest, she was there every step of the way with great editing and wise counsel. Her encouragement to keep the heart and humor in the first edition made all the difference, and I am forever grateful for her help.

Others came along to help as the book progressed. Clarissa Pinkola Estés appeared at just the right moment with her kind-hearted support and good words. She is truly *la madrina*, the spiritual godmother of this book.

Jennifer Woodhull, wordsmith supreme and faithful friend, added her considerable skills to both editions. For this latest one, she stepped in with helpful last-minute editing and an invaluable consultation on what the duck should say.

I also appreciate the good editing skills of Nancy Adess, who brought her keen eye for organization and clarity to the second edition and soothed my writer's nerves with her steadiness and good humor.

David Payne, my patient editor at Lippincott Williams & Wilkins, was always there with useful opinions and clear answers to my endless questions.

The artist, Dolph Smith, was most generous in allowing me to use his beautiful work for the book's cover. I so appreciate his kind support and especially all the time he spent rummaging through his files to find a transparency we could use. Thanks to Kathy Albers, owner of the piece, for graciously allowing us to use this wonderful collage. The graphic artists, Amy Sharp and Kelli Glazier Smith, designed the appealing front cover and interior design, respectively, for the first edition. Others who helped by tidying up the manuscript the first time around were Jennifer Cook, Anne Hoff, Jennifer Werner, and Ben Bledsoe.

Many others added their talents and knowledge to the first edition. My smart friend Suzanne Henley came up with the idea of using artwork on the cover. Les Kertay contributed the useful concept of specialness as a red flag. At a critical stage, Karen Craig helped me define my audience. Diane Bauer Sable is the good massage therapist that my friend Robbie McQuiston praises in Chapter 3. Carol Risher and Bonnie Gintis added helpful information.

Many thanks to Leslie Young, editor-in-chief of *Massage & Bodywork* magazine, who generously allowed me to use passages from my column and cartoon ideas similar to Mari's cartoons that ran with the column. I also thank her for allowing me leeway on *M&B* deadlines when book deadlines were looming and, mostly, for being a joy to work with.

Over the years, I've been blessed to have compassionate and skilled bodywork teachers to inspire me. In the world of Rolfing, they were Peter Melchior, Tom Wing, and the late great Stacey Mills.

The dedicated and highly talented staff of the Rosen Method Center Southwest in Santa Fe showed me what miracles could happen when you take care with boundaries. Thanks to Sandra Wooten, Cameron Hough, and Julia Martin, whose life-changing workshops inspired me to start writing the first edition. Every bodyworker needs a loving community of colleagues, and they have been mine.

I'm also grateful to my thoughtful and caring colleagues who contributed useful information and personal experiences. Some who helped out especially were Keith Eric Grant, Brian H. Thayer, Douglas L. Barhorst, and Sheryl Rapée-Adams. Special thanks to my entire online bodywork forum for challenging me to think, making me laugh, and renewing my faith in the profession.

Other colleagues who helped were Jack Blackburn, who offered expert knowledge about supervision and supervision groups. Thanks also to Holly B. White for her contribution.

Much gratitude for my friends who stood beside me and sometimes offered great stories to use: Ellen Klyce, Jill Breslau, Charlotte Schultz, Helen Luce, Dana Siler, and, of course, Ferdie. My talented cousin Ellen Rolfes has been a constant cheering section, as have my brother John and sister-in-law Margaret.

Everyone needs angels. During the writing of these two editions, the angels that celebrated my best efforts and carried me through the hard times were Janet Zimmerman, Karen McCaulley, and Cindy Westcott. I appreciate all that I learned from these wise and kind women.

For this edition, there were respected colleagues who read the early drafts and offered thoughtful and valuable feedback that I took to heart. I thank them all for their time and conscientious efforts. Their names appear on the reviewers' page.

For the first edition, I interviewed many experienced and outstanding manual therapists and asked others to give me feedback about chapters in progress. Those good people were: Rob Bauer, Ben Benjamin, Kathryn Benson, Mary Bernau-Eigen, Heida Brenneke, Sue Brenner, Rose Bronec,

Gary Brownlee, Sharon Burch,, Carol Burke, Marie Carbone, Olivia Cheever, Daphne Chellos, Melissa Chipman, Amrita Daigle, Kirsten DeMier, Barbara Tift Featherstone, Alan Fogel, Linda Frisone, Sandy Fritz, Cindy Getchonis, William J. Greenberg, Karna Handy, Annie Hartzog, Natasha Heifitz, Joseph Heller, Sabrina Johnson, Anna Johnson-Chase, Arnold Katz, Les Kertay, Robert K. King, Carole LaRochelle, David Lauterstein, Lucy Liben, Marcy Lindheimer, Til Luchau, Michael Maskornick, Edward W. Maupin, Leslee McKnight-McCallum, Heather Merritt, Margaret Avery Moon, Thomas Myers, Rebecca Naifeh, Laurie Owen, Jim Pearson, Lee Phillips, Dianne Polseno, Marion Rosen, Paul Rubin, Vivien Schapera, Bill Scholl, Jan Schwartz, Ethel Scrivener, Kristina Shaw, Chris Smith, Cherie Sohnen-Moe, Gail Stewart, Theresa E. Stogner, Kylea Taylor, Diana L. Thompson, Angela Watkins, Nancy Forst Williamson, Charles Wiltsie, Chloe Wing, Sandra Wooten, and Dwight Zieman.

REVIEWERS

Thomas R. Filippi, MA, MS
School of Massage Therapy,
    Morgantown Beauty College
Morgantown, West Virginia

Richard Greely, MEd, LMT
Assistant Professor, Columbus State
    Community College
Columbus, Ohio

Sue Mapel, LICSW
Dean of Students, Muscular
    Therapy Institute
Cambridge, Massachusetts

**Pamela Rose, BA, PIDP
(Education), DipAdult
(Community and Higher
Education)**
Education Director, Okanagan
    Valley College of Massage
    Therapy
Vernon, British Columbia, Canada

Frank Schwartz, BA, MS, LMT
Harmony Path School of Massage
    Therapy
Rocky River, Ohio

CONTENTS

ABOUT THE AUTHOR . . . . *vii*

FOREWORD . . . . *ix*

PREFACE . . . . *xi*

ACKNOWLEDGMENTS . . . . *xv*

REVIEWERS . . . . *xix*

Chapter 1: THE EDUCATED HEART: THE NEED FOR
PROFESSIONAL BOUNDARIES 1

Chapter 2: PROTECTIVE CIRCLES: BOUNDARIES AND THE
PROFESSIONAL RELATIONSHIP 12

Chapter 3: FRAMEWORK: NUTS AND BOLTS OF BOUNDARIES 25

Chapter 4: CLIENT-PRACTITIONER DYNAMICS: BOUNDARIES
AND THE POWER IMBALANCE 46

Chapter 5: ETHICAL BOUNDARIES: FROM THEORY TO PRACTICE . . . 64

Chapter 6: BOUNDARIES AND THE POWER OF WORDS 84

Chapter 7: SEXUAL BOUNDARIES: PROTECTING OUR CLIENTS 100

Chapter 8: SEXUAL BOUNDARIES: PROTECTING OURSELVES 115

Chapter 9: FINANCIAL BOUNDARIES: GETTING COMFORTABLE . . . 131
WITH MONEY

Chapter 10: DUAL RELATIONSHIPS AND BOUNDARIES: WEARING
MANY HATS 146

Chapter 11: HELP WITH BOUNDARIES: SUPPORT, CONSULTATION,
AND SUPERVISION 160

Appendix A: AMERICAN MASSAGE THERAPY ASSOCIATION CODE
OF ETHICS 173

Appendix B: ASSOCIATED BODYWORK AND MASSAGE
PROFESSIONALS CODE OF ETHICS 174

Appendix C: RELATED READINGS 177

GLOSSARY 179

INDEX 183

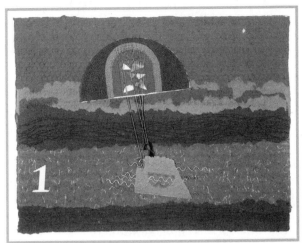

Chapter 1

*T*HE EDUCATED HEART: THE NEED FOR PROFESSIONAL BOUNDARIES

Our profession is still young. We are still exploring what it means to be a good **manual therapist**. We are learning that technical skill is only one aspect of a responsible and successful practice. For our work to be effective, we need solid professional relationships with our clients. We create such relationships by knowing what belongs in our interactions with our clients and what doesn't. Clients will appreciate our friendliness and warmth. But more than that, clients need the security of sturdy professional boundaries.

Our work is unusually personal. To most people, what we do is unfamiliar, and the intimacy of the work can stir up deep emotional associations. We make this potentially confusing and highly charged situation safe for our clients and for ourselves by maintaining professional boundaries.

Attention to boundaries is also the key to a smoothly running practice. When we create a safe environment, our clients settle in and go deeper. Our work lives flow more smoothly. We have more satisfied clients who come back and who tell their friends about us. We have fewer difficult clients and more clients who leave our offices with a lighter heart and a lighter step.

Most of us come to this work with good intentions and a genuine wish to serve others. These aspirations flourish best within the structure of good professional boundaries. To truly serve our clients, we need not just good hearts, but educated hearts.

Manual therapists: Trained professionals who touch the physical or energetic body of the client or who use a method of movement to affect the body of a client for the purpose of facilitating awareness, health, and well-being. As used here, the term is interchangeable with somatic practitioners and includes massage therapists, bodyworkers, movement educators, practitioners of Oriental methods, and practitioners who work primarily with energy fields.

The Need for Educated Boundaries

When we hear the word "professional," we may think of a clinical atmosphere or a distant and aloof therapist. But professionalism doesn't mean acting stuffy or keeping our clients at arm's length. It simply means that, when we're working, our focus is on our clients. We pay attention to them; we're sensitive to their vulnerability. Being professional is just an educated way of being kind.

The best way we can demonstrate this kindness is by keeping appropriate **boundaries**. Clients instinctively feel safer when we set clear boundaries. Maintaining good boundaries is also a kindness to practitioners. Not only do we feel more secure when expectations are clear, but also our work is more rewarding.

Boundaries:
In this context, a boundary is like a protective circle around the professional relationship that separates what is appropriate within that relationship from what is not.

Understanding the Need for Boundaries

The success of our practices depends, to a large extent, on how we handle our professional relationships. No matter how technically skilled we may be, our clients won't get the full benefits of our work if they don't feel safe with us. A casual attitude toward boundaries can jar clients and make them uneasy. When people complain about a manual therapy session they received, their complaint is not usually about the practitioner's inadequate effleurage or inability to name all the muscles in the foot. Instead, they'll say, "She talked about her boyfriend the whole hour" or "I felt nervous going to a bodyworker who works out of a bedroom in his house."

To understand why safe boundaries are crucial, we have to be aware of the special circumstances of our work, particularly the physical intimacy, the effects of touch, and the power dynamic in our relationships with clients.

Keeping Clients Safe

Much of the public does not have a clear idea of what we do, how we are trained, and what to expect from us. They may associate our work with the sexual overtones of massage parlors. They may be wary of our lack of traditional medical credentials or fear that we will injure them or make a physical problem worse. It is up to us to make the situation a safe one in which they can relax and heal. It is up to us to show that we are serious about what we do and that we are genuinely concerned about our clients' welfare. Maintaining appropriate professional boundaries is a crucial step in setting the right tone for safety.

For us, the intimacy of our work is something we can take for granted. It can be easy to forget how scary and potentially intrusive some clients may find physical touch. We live in a culture in which touch is often experienced as leading to seduction or violence. For many people, accidentally brushing up against someone they don't know is uncomfortable. Yet in our work, clients agree to be touched by a relative stranger, usually while the client is naked or only partially clothed. Some clients may fear our negative judgments about their physical appearance. In a society obsessed with being trim and blemish free, clients are revealing their less-than-perfect bodies to us. No wonder some people have a hard time letting go.

Uncovered Feelings and Memories

Touch can bring up long-buried feelings and memories that clients may find both surprising and frightening. Even in the most caring of families, certain feelings or aspects of ourselves can meet with disapproval from those around us. As children, we unconsciously learn to hold back these feelings. We may also protect ourselves by blocking out unpleasant or traumatic memories. Without being conscious of it, we may hide uncomfortable experiences or emotions—perhaps even from ourselves.

When we hold back our feelings, aspects of ourselves, or memories, we literally hold them back with our muscles. What is held back can get locked into our tissue, creating tension. This is true whether the holding began last week or decades ago. When clients are touched, especially as their muscles relax, those memories and feelings may emerge.

> After her massage therapist loosens up her tight shoulder muscles, a client suddenly remembers last week's argument with her boss and how angry she felt.

> A 60-year-old client tells his massage therapist that he's never had any injuries. However, when his bodyworker works with his lower leg, memories come flooding back of falling out of a tree and spraining his ankle when he was 10 years old. As if it were yesterday, the client remembers how it happened, how his father reacted, and how scared he felt.

> A client cries as subtle shifts in her pelvis facilitated by her movement educator reawaken the long-buried nightmare of the months she spent in a punitive home for unwed mothers 20 years earlier.

Clients bring all of their held-back memories and feelings to the table, usually without realizing it. Although many clients come to us only for relaxation and can easily appreciate the simple pleasure of being touched without having such memories intrude, others who have experienced trauma may have a more difficult time letting go. Most often, clients won't become aware of suppressed feelings during the session; however, they may express those feelings in unconscious ways. For instance, a client who was physically or sexually abused may be wary of his practitioner or expect to be harmed without knowing why. Even if potentially scary or unpleasant material doesn't emerge, our touch may nudge the edge of it. We can't judge by superficial appearances how emotionally fragile any one client might be. Because of that, we need to provide safe and reassuring boundaries for *all* our clients.

Acknowledging Power and Responsibility

The dynamics of the client-practitioner relationship are complex and often subtle. Our clients automatically give us more power than they would, for instance, if they met us on the street. They are often looking to us to alleviate their physical or emotional stress or discomfort, which puts them in a vulnerable and often dependent position. Consequently, our words and actions tend to carry more weight and authority for them. Even though they may not be conscious of it, we can become bigger in their eyes—more like a doctor or parent figure. Clients may put us on a pedestal, thinking we can do no wrong. For practitioners, our relationship with clients brings with it built-in authority and responsibilities. Our task is to meet our clients' vulnerability with respect and kindness, and we do that by maintaining secure boundaries.

Seven Common Misconceptions About Boundaries

As much as we want to be respectful and kind, many somatic practitioners haven't been trained in either the whys or the how-tos of being professional. The dynamics of the professional relationship can be intricate, and the best course of action is not always clear. We may not even realize some of the mistakes that have arisen from our lack of education and awareness.

Some errors are more serious than others. Probably no client will haul us into court for talking too much during the session about the movie we saw last night, but discussing a client's problems with an outsider could land us in front of an ethics committee. Sometimes we can't gauge how big a problem our boundary mistake will be. The client who heard too much about last night's movie may not sue, but he may decide not to come back. Then again, he might be a long-time client who forgives the disruption of his relaxation—this time.

Some of us have learned about the importance of good boundaries through painful experience. Here's what a colleague said:

> A couple of years into my practice, I realized it was a mess. Clients became friends, friends became clients, and I was putting a good deal of energy into sorting it out. Sometimes sessions became social visits, and my clients weren't able to get the full benefits of the work. Sometimes friends who had become clients didn't want to pay my usual fees or respect my time. It helped a lot when I started being firmer about boundaries. When I stopped socializing during sessions, clients were able to settle down and take in the work, and when I became clearer about what I expected and expressed those expectations to my clients, friends stopped taking advantage of me.

Because our profession is a relatively new one, many of us have had to piece together our own ideas of professional conduct without the benefit of specific training or education in that aspect of our practice. As a result, some common misconceptions have been born out of understandable confusion.

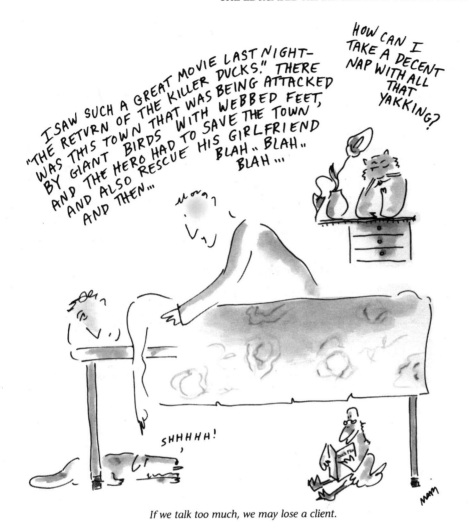

I SAW SUCH A GREAT MOVIE LAST NIGHT— "THE RETURN OF THE KILLER DUCKS." THERE WAS THIS TOWN THAT WAS BEING ATTACKED BY GIANT BIRDS WITH WEBBED FEET, AND THE HERO HAD TO SAVE THE TOWN AND ALSO RESCUE HIS GIRLFRIEND BLAH .. BLAH .. BLAH ... AND THEN ...

HOW CAN I TAKE A DECENT NAP WITH ALL THAT YAKKING?

SHHHHH!

If we talk too much, we may lose a client.

Clarifying these misconceptions can help remove any doubts about the importance of healthy professional boundaries.

Misconception #1: "I want to be natural with clients; boundaries create barriers."

This concern about maintaining appropriate boundaries comes in many forms, such as, "I want to be authentic with my clients," and "I don't want to put myself above my clients." This is often how we justify talking about our own issues with clients or letting them see the off-duty side of us, confiding to them and complaining to them as if they were friends.

However, being professional means that we are careful about what we reveal to our clients, not out of a sense of superiority, but out of a wish to keep the focus on the client. When we share personal information with clients, they may feel obligated to take care of us in the way that friends tend to do for each other. At the least, it takes attention away from the reason they are there—to have *us* pay attention to their needs. It's misguided to think that letting our hair down with clients is always therapeutic for them. When we are tempted to complain about our love lives, share our political beliefs, or tell clients how tired we are, we have to stop and wonder how that will add to their feelings of security.

In rare instances, it can be helpful to let clients know that we, too, have struggled with the same kinds of issues. If we know a client well, we might want to reassure or inspire her by remarking that we once had the same problem. However, such sharing should be carefully thought out. Unless clients already respect us and know our strength, talking about our struggles could make them question our capabilities, expect less of us, or feel obliged to help us. For the same reasons, we should only mention issues that we have already resolved, not current problems.

The truth is that we do have more power in our relationships with clients; recognizing that fact is being responsible, not arrogant. But having good boundaries doesn't mean that we can't be genuinely caring people in our practices. Authenticity is reassuring and appropriate when we are down to earth in how we present ourselves, when we do not mystify what we are doing or pretend to be all knowing. It can be healing to allow clients to see the compassion we feel toward them. We can, for instance, let clients see that their stories have touched us, and we can sympathize with them about their concerns—but it's not appropriate to ask them to do the same for us.

Boundaries aren't elitist or intended to make a client feel "less than" us or disrespected. Quite the opposite; boundaries are a gift to clients.

Misconception #2: "I'll just use my common sense."

We may think that professional boundaries are just common sense, but it's not that simple. Making good judgments doesn't necessarily come naturally. After we've practiced long enough, we can begin to look and feel like naturals, but that's not the same as "just being ourselves" or only using common sense.

Without clear, thought-out guidelines, our decisions about boundaries and ethics are likely to be based on a hodgepodge of conflicting influences. We are affected by what our upbringing has taught us about pain, dependency, sex, and intimacy. We're swayed by our own biases and prejudices. Our judgment can be clouded by our egos and by the all-too-human need to be in control, right, or important. Or we may imitate mentors and teachers who themselves didn't understand the need for good boundaries. We may rely on advice from our friends or partners. And when in doubt, we may throw in a random piece of wisdom from the latest self-help book we've read.

If, for instance, our own boundaries have been violated as children—sexually, emotionally or physically—then what comes "naturally" to us may be off-kilter.

To make good judgment calls, we need to know ourselves well. Unless we are self-aware, our personal histories or trauma can interfere with making wise choices. If, for instance, our own boundaries have been violated as children—sexually, emotionally or physically—then what comes "naturally" to us may be off-kilter.

We all have blind spots that interfere with our effectiveness. Even if we have had no significant childhood trauma, we bring to our work all of our personal history. We have rough patches in our behavior where we do things that don't make sense or fail to see what's in front of us. We may deny, rationalize, and project the things we dislike about ourselves onto other people. That is part of human nature.

> After gaining unwanted weight, a colleague found himself mentally judging his overweight clients. When he realized what he was doing and how it was related to his judgment about his own extra pounds, he was able to address and eventually change his negative feelings.

> A massage therapist with a history of being sexually abused by a relative routinely overlapped her social and her professional lives, often urging people she found attractive to come to her for massage so that she could get to know them better. Until she sought professional help, she didn't realize the connection between how her abuser had overstepped family boundaries and how she was overstepping boundaries in her practice. Because being careless with boundaries felt familiar to her, she hadn't been aware that it was a problem.

None of us is perfect, but it's our responsibility to learn what professional boundaries are and maintain them. Good boundaries are too crucial to leave to just our common sense.

Misconception #3: "I've learned technique, and that's all I need to know."

Until recently, medical schools focused on teaching only anatomy and medical techniques, as if human relationships with patients don't matter. Perhaps, without thinking, we have used that same model in our profession. Until recently, many of our own schools have stressed anatomy and technique, ignoring the importance of relationship dynamics. Although that omission is understandable, it's important that we now realize that there's more to our work than physical mechanics. It's heartening to see that many massage and manual therapy schools (along with many medical schools) have added courses on boundaries, ethics, relationship dynamics, and the importance of a healing alliance between practitioner and client. In general, we're moving past the idea that a client is simply a mass of muscles to be manipulated.

As manual therapists, we may need to pay even more attention to boundaries than doctors do. People don't expect to be able to let go and have a blissful, transcendent experience in a doctor's treatment room. But when people come to us, they are hoping to be able to drop their defenses. They want to leave feeling more centered, more alive, more themselves. To set the stage for that experience, we need a good deal more education and training than just learning the name of the erector spinae, for example. No technique, no matter how state of the art it is, can ensure that a client will trust us. (Impeccable boundaries will not ensure trust either, but they will improve the odds.)

How people heal is a mystery. Humans are a complicated mix of psyche, spirit, body, and emotions, and we can't really know where one of those elements stops and another begins. We can learn a hundred new techniques and still not understand why people hurt. But we can create an atmosphere within which healing can take place.

Misconception #4: "I don't need to know anything about psychological dynamics; I'm not a psychotherapist."

Some of us feel it's not our business to try to understand our relationships with our clients. Perhaps we fear that it will lead to "playing psychologist" with clients or trying to analyze them.

We're right to avoid analyzing clients' psychological problems and airing our opinions—that would be intrusive and a violation of boundaries. However, it is very much our business to learn how to create a safe emotional environment for our clients. And we can do that without inappropriately dabbling in psychological counseling.

All health care professionals could probably benefit from knowing more about their relationships with clients. Only by understanding the more hidden dimensions of the client-practitioner relationship can we have a deeper appreciation for the vulnerability of clients and their need for safety. We don't have to be psychotherapists to want to be sensitive to our clients' needs.

Misconception #5: "I have needs, too."

> A massage therapist who canceled a session at the last minute to attend to minor personal business didn't appreciate why her client was so upset. The therapist said, "My clients have to understand that I have needs, too."

Of course that massage therapist has personal needs—we all do. But it's inappropriate to allow those needs to interfere with our work. We're there to

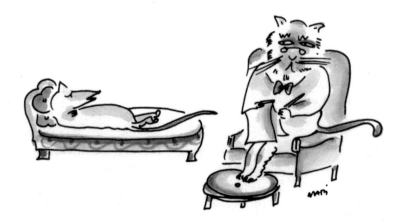

focus on our clients' needs, which means putting our personal lives aside. Although we cannot avoid the occasional intrusion of a personal situation into our work, we have to realize that being professional means that the show must go on and, when it cannot, we let our clients down. (We can consider offering a free session when we are forced to cancel without the standard 24 hours notice.)

At the same time, it's perfectly fine, and even desirable, to be concerned with our *professional* needs. We should ask our clients to treat us as professionals and respect our professional boundaries. For instance, we have a right to ask our clients to arrive on time, pay at each session, and give adequate cancellation notice.

Sometimes we have difficulty setting boundaries to protect ourselves. We may routinely allow clients to cancel at the last minute without paying for the session, or we may frequently give a full session to a client who arrives 20 minutes late. Allowing clients to take advantage of us can lead to resentment on our part and confusion on the part of the client.

Professional boundaries define the relationship as having limits and standards that both practitioner and client respect. These standards benefit both parties by helping everyone feel more secure in what is a uniquely intimate situation.

Misconception #6: "My connection with my clients is through the healing energy in my hands, and that's what's important."

Having "healing energy" is a good start, but is it enough? Our work is intuitive, and sometimes our hands feel magically drawn to just the right place. We can have a subtle connection with our clients that is hard to define. But that isn't all there is to it. If we get too caught up in the mystery of our work, we can overlook our clients' basic needs. We can gaze into the distance with misty eyes and speak of our magical connection with our clients, but if that is our only focus, our clients will be wondering why the room is so cold, why we were 10 minutes late, and why we keep forgetting what their names are.

Misconception #7: "But I know practitioners who are careless about boundaries and still have successful practices."

In a certain respect, this statement isn't completely a misconception. It's true that there are practitioners with successful practices who disregard many professional standards and boundary concerns—maybe they frequently make friends of their clients, they're careless about confidentiality, or their offices are a mess. Most of these are well-meaning practitioners who never learned the importance of good boundaries. They benefit from the fact that clients will forgive a great deal if a practitioner has a good heart and "good hands." A careful look at their practices, however, generally reveals that they could make their clients much happier and their work lives much easier by paying closer attention to professional boundaries.

> A successful practitioner gave a great massage but always started her sessions late. As her clients waited on the table sometimes 5 or 10 minutes, they could hear her making phone calls or talking with her business partner. Although many of her clients were annoyed, few said anything. The practitioner noticed how hard she had to work to help her clients relax and trust her at the beginning of each massage, but she didn't realize how much her own behavior contributed to their tension.

Coming of Age

Good boundaries don't occur naturally. They need to be studied and practiced in the same way that we learn anatomy, physiology, or technique. The art of setting boundaries is the intangible element that brings out the best in both practitioner and client.

Although setting clear boundaries may, at first glance, seem to distance us from our clients, the opposite is actually true. Good boundaries don't create walls between client and practitioner; rather, they create a safe space within which we can touch clients' hearts and ease their spirits.

QUESTIONS FOR REFLECTION

1. In as much detail as you can, remember a particularly great massage you have had as a client or imagine what one would be like. What elements made it (would make it) a great experience? Are all of these elements related to the practitioner's knowledge of technique and anatomy? How many components are related to the professional atmosphere and the attitude of the practitioner?

2. Have you ever experienced a release of feelings and memories during a bodywork session or a massage? If it's hard to conceptualize how emotions and memories can be stored in our bodies, try this exercise: The next time you receive a massage, observe the thoughts and feelings that float through your mind during the session. Consider how your thoughts and feelings during a session may be related to the tension and holding in your body that are being released.

3. Misconception #1 is about the concern that keeping professional boundaries leads to a less natural relationship with clients. Think about what has been true for you as a client or a patient. Has a health professional (doctor, chiropractor, massage therapist, other bodyworker) ever been casual with you or self-revealing in a way that wasn't helpful? Has the opposite ever been true for you—that a health profes-

sional's behavior wasn't strictly professional, but you found it to be helpful? If you've experienced both of these, what made the one helpful and the other not?

4. As you were growing up, did you come to believe anything about pain, dependency, or intimacy that might interfere with your having a non-judgmental attitude toward your clients? For instance, perhaps you were brought up to believe that only weaklings complain when they are hurting. How would that belief affect your attitude toward clients who (appropriately) tell you about their aches and pains? How might you unlearn attitudes that aren't useful to you as a manual therapist?

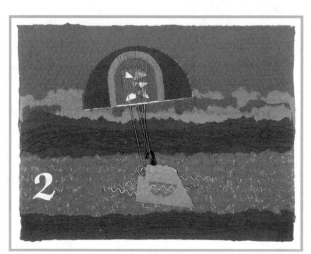

Chapter 2

PROTECTIVE CIRCLES: BOUNDARIES AND THE PROFESSIONAL RELATIONSHIP

Professional therapeutic relationship: A relationship between client and practitioner that is focused on the well-being of the client.

Contract: An agreement between practitioner and client that is often implied rather than explicit about what each will or will not do. An ethical contract must be within the bounds of the practitioner's training and the ethical standards of her or his profession. The client agrees to give specific fees, goods, or services in return and agrees to be respectful of the practitioner's guidelines for appropriate behavior.

Boundaries are like protective circles surrounding the professional relationship. Rather than being barriers that separate us from our clients, good boundaries safeguard both practitioner and client. Boundaries separate what is appropriate in professional relationships from what is not. When used well, boundaries clarify limits and expectations, helping to keep both client and practitioner secure.

In theory, the idea of staying within professional boundaries may sound simple. The client comes to us for massage therapy, bodywork, or movement education. We do what we are trained to do and what we have contracted to do. The client pays us an agreed-upon amount or completes a pre-arranged trade. Although this may not sound complicated, it can be all too easy to lose our focus and overstep these boundaries. In understanding how to establish healthy boundaries, we need to consider first our role in the **therapeutic relationship**.

Understanding Our Professional Role

Taking on a role does not mean that we pretend; rather, it means that during our interactions with clients, we behave in ways that are appropriate to the **therapeutic contract**. The contract is determined by what we have been trained to do and, more importantly, by what the client is paying us to do. We may have training in clinical psychology, for instance, but if clients are coming to us for accupressure, we should not take on the role of psychological counselor.

We always have two roles with our clients: a specific role as a certain kind of somatic practitioner and a more general role as a professional. The first role—and the one most commonly recognized—is the role defined by our specific training, such as massage therapist, Feldenkrais teacher, or Trager practitioner. In this role, we use a certain method of massage therapy, bodywork, or movement education to help a client. The broader role that we must learn is that of a professional person—this is the role that has been traditionally neglected and that can cause the most confusion. When we take on a professional role, for example, we keep our personal lives, opinions, and needs out of our sessions. Also, as part of that role, we expect to be treated as a professional with all that it entails.

To have a solid and rewarding practice, every somatic practitioner needs to be comfortable in these two roles—both as a certain type of practitioner and as a professional. However, learning to be at ease with our roles takes time. We may be able to learn a couple of massage strokes in a weekend, but it takes a much longer time to develop a solid sense of ourselves as professional somatic practitioners.

The Professional Therapeutic Relationship—What Stays In

If boundaries form a protective circle around the professional therapeutic relationship, what is reasonable to include in that circle? Here is a brief description of the most basic elements of the professional therapeutic relationship, all of which are discussed more fully in later chapters.

Client-Centered Actions and Words

The concept of being "client-centered" is central to the therapeutic relationship. "Client-centered" means that our actions and words should be motivated by what is best for the client. Being client-centered means that we put aside our personal egos, interests and needs, likes and dislikes and act in the best interests of the client. At the same time, this doesn't mean that "the customer is always right" or that we should let clients take advantage of us. After all, it's also in our clients' best interests to provide them with clear limits.

Being client-centered means, for one thing, that clients have a right to ask for what they want. We don't want to become dictators, ordering clients to be quiet if we decide they're talking too much or becoming upset if they dare to ask us to vary our massage routine for their comfort. Clients need to be free to make requests as long as the requests are not abusive, destructive, or inappropriate. They should be encouraged to make their needs and wishes known. When clients do speak up, it's our job either to adjust and meet their needs or explain why what they are requesting is not appropriate, in their best interests, or within the scope of our training or abilities.

> A practitioner complained about a client: "When I came back into the room after giving her time to get undressed and on the table, she had taken all the pillows in the room and arranged them around her on the table—under her knees and her neck and different places."

In this story, one wonders why the therapist is complaining: it sounds as if the client is doing the practitioner's job for her. Unless the client was destroying property, there's no reason why she shouldn't make herself comfortable.

There are instances when we would not want to adjust to clients' wishes or automatically honor their requests. If the client's arrangement of pillows might interfere with the session in some way, the practitioner could always explain why the arrangement needs to be altered and ask the client's permission to make the change. Or, for instance, if a client has a pain in his neck and asks that we spend the whole hour working on his neck, we might want to suggest that because neck pain often reflects tension throughout the body, he might receive greater benefit from a more complete massage.

Confidentiality

Confidentiality is at the core of professional relationships. It begins with the first phone call and continues for the entirety of the relationship.

If we want to be respected as professionals, we have to honor our clients' privacy and confidentiality. We cannot gossip about what they said, complain about what they did, brag about how much they liked our work, or in any way discuss or relate what clients said or did during our sessions (or during any professional contact). Confidentiality is at the core of professional relationships. It begins with the first phone call and continues for the entirety of the relationship.

A friend relates this breach of confidentiality:

> I recently received a massage from a practitioner I hadn't been to before. I was surprised when she began telling me how one of her clients, a man we both knew, was responding well to her work. She talked about the physical problems he had had and what relief he'd gotten from her massage. I think I was supposed to be impressed by this report, but all it did was make me uncomfortable. I thought, "What will she say about me to other people?"

Consistency

When asked what keeps clients coming back, many experienced therapists put consistency high on their list. Clients are reassured by consistency and reliability (assuming that we are consistently good about professional standards and not, for instance, consistently flaky or insensitive). After clients have gotten used to our settings and styles, they can be rattled by changes in routine, in the office space, in session times, and any other part of our work with them. For instance, if a client has a regular time slot, it's important to try to keep that time slot for him and not move him to a different time. If we do have to move our office or change a regular client's hour, we can be careful to keep other elements of our work the same. Clients can trust us if we are consistently attentive and professional, and they can relax more deeply if they can trust us.

Informed Consent and Right of Refusal

Informed consent is a formal term meaning that clients have a right to understand all that is involved in our work with them, and we must have their educated, informed consent in order for our work with them to be ethical. It means that there should be no surprises for our clients.

As much as possible, we should spell out verbally and in writing our contracts with clients. They need to know what our training is, what methods we will be using, and the possible benefits and risks of those methods. We also have to let clients know that they can ask us to stop at any time and for any reason. They have what is formally called the right of refusal. It's never appropriate for us to be impatient or annoyed by clients who question our work or credentials or who don't want to take part in any aspect of our work. Clients need to know that we are offering our expertise but that they are ultimately in control of the session.

Our Rights as Professionals

Along with spelling out to clients what they can expect from our work and getting their consent, we need to be clear about what we expect of them. Upholding our rights as professionals is an important basic principle for a healthy therapeutic relationship. We can, for instance, expect our clients to show up on time and leave when sessions are done. We can expect them to give us adequate cancellation notice and pay our fees on time. We should not work with abusive or disrespectful clients, and, indeed, we can decline to work with any client when we do not feel it is in our or their best interests to do so. (However, we need to be familiar with the codes of practice in our state or, in Canada, in our province that pertain to refusal to work with a client. Those who work for a spa or for another professional also need to know their employer's standards on this question.)

The Professional Therapeutic Relationship— What Stays Out

As somatic practitioners, we have to stay within the limits of our scope of practice, that is, the traditional knowledge base and standard practices of the profession. Staying inside those boundaries sometimes requires us to walk a fine line. Is it psychological counseling when we comfort a recently divorced client? Are we giving medical advice when we suggest that a client might not

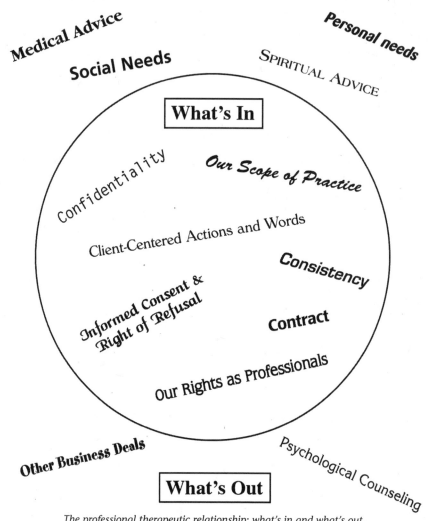

The professional therapeutic relationship: what's in and what's out.

need his shoe lift anymore? When are we overstepping the line between friend and client? When are we giving too much personal information?

It's fair to assume that every somatic practitioner has violated boundaries, if only in some small way. Keeping good boundaries is a little like steering a car—it takes constant correction. Just when we think we're on a smooth path, we hit a bump. It's not a question of whether we make mistakes; we're human and we're bound to make mistakes. It's more a question of knowing when we've made mistakes and then being willing to change our behavior.

> A colleague who often gave advice to an unhappily married client realized that he was in over his head. He told the client he would gladly continue to be a sympathetic ear for her, but if she wanted to work on changing her relationship with her husband, he would help her find a good marriage counselor.

A bodyworker became aware that when he talked too much during a session, he literally would have a bad taste in his mouth. Now when he gets that taste, he knows it's time to be quiet.

After a too-short vacation, a colleague realized she was dragging in just a few minutes late to all her sessions. As soon as she noticed this, she began making extra efforts to be on time and to take better care of herself.

The challenge is to be aware of boundaries and value them, yet be tolerant of our own imperfection. However, because our mistakes are usually at the client's expense and can hurt our practices, we don't want to be too tolerant of our shortcomings.

There are three common ways that we venture outside the safe boundaries of the professional relationship: bringing in our social and personal needs, going outside our scope of practice and expertise, and mixing our practices with other businesses. Here is a brief overview to highlight these major problem areas. All of these areas are discussed in more detail in later chapters.

Social Needs and Personal Needs

Perhaps the most frequent boundary confusion is between our professional lives and our social lives. Ways that we can overstep those boundaries range from the relatively harmless, such as an occasional lapse into chatting during a session, to the more problematic, such as socializing with clients, to the downright unethical, such as dating a client.

Some of us don't understand why it's important to draw a boundary between our social lives and our professional ones. What's wrong with having a casual conversation with a client during a session or even sharing something personal about ourselves with our clients? What's wrong with a friendly cup of tea? Maybe nothing is, but these actions can often take advantage of clients' vulnerability or interfere with their receiving the full benefits of their sessions.

Our boundary slip-ups usually have an innocent motivation. Here are some common reasons that we may want to bring our social needs into our professional lives.

THE NEED FOR SOCIAL INTERACTION

Probably the most common complaint clients have is about practitioners who talk too much. Clients are trying to relax and drift away into their own world, and we keep pulling them out of that world with our demands for their attention. Clients rarely ask us to be quiet. They won't say, "I don't want to hear another word about your new car." Clients are both too polite and too influenced by the power imbalance inherent in the relationship.

Rather than asking us to stop talking, they usually respond politely and then perhaps complain to their friends—or worse, not come back.

THE NEED FOR FRIENDS

Some practitioners may say their clients are like friends. We may be on friendly terms with our clients, but are they really like our friends? Do we have friends who come to see us and immediately throw off their clothes and describe all their aches and pains?

There's a difference between a client and a friend. (And if our friend becomes our client, then the client role comes first during the session hour.) Personal friends put up with our lapses and our flaws; they listen patiently while we go on for 10 minutes about what somebody said to us and what we said back. They can let us know—and forgive us—when we hurt their feelings. Friends aren't paying us.

As soon as someone becomes a client, we need to be aware of our therapeutic role, both in and out of sessions. The more we muddy the waters between the social and the professional, the more likely we are to do or say something that will interfere with having a professional, healing relationship.

> A female bodyworker used a male client's sessions to lament the woes of her divorce and the problems of being single. This was confusing to the client—he wondered if she wanted a romantic relationship with him. When he asked her out on a date, however, she refused him. He felt hurt and rejected and stopped making appointments with her.

This client ended up feeling wounded or betrayed by a relationship that should have been therapeutic. We usually cheat our clients when we put the focus on ourselves, when we ask them to listen to us and take care of us.

THE NEED FOR ROMANCE AND EXCITEMENT

There's another reason to avoid the temptation to socialize with our clients. Let's be honest—when the wish to socialize is there, isn't it sometimes because we're attracted to that client? Perhaps the client has a crush on us that we are enjoying. If we socialize with that client, what kind of message are we sending? Even if we are not flirting, the client may think we are. Because it's unethical to date clients or even to flirt with them, we'd be better off keeping the relationship strictly professional—and seeking outside advice or discontinuing our work with a client for whom there is a strong attraction.

Some of us can't avoid social interactions with clients. Those of us who live in small towns or are involved with small communities within a large town may have a difficult time keeping that boundary firm. We may frequently run into clients at outside events, friends and acquaintances may become clients, or clients may become friends. How to navigate these different relationships is discussed more fully in Chapter 10 on dual relationships.

Going Outside Our Scope of Practice or Expertise

We go outside boundaries when we make exaggerated claims about the effects of our methods or when we behave as if we are experts in areas in which we either have no training or only a relatively small amount of training. For instance, we are on thin ice if we guarantee that massage will lower a client's cholesterol level. Likewise, if we tell clients what foods to eat or why they should divorce their spouses, we have ventured into territory for which we have neither training nor contract.

Perhaps the wish to inflate our work comes from the general insecurity of the profession. We don't live in a culture where ads on the bus read "Got aches and pains? Consult your bodyworker first." The benefits of our work are becoming more widely known, but many people still don't know how it can help them. For the most part, the manual therapies are still unacknowledged by a culture accustomed to a traditional medical viewpoint. For many of us, there is a vast gap between what we know to be the value of our work and the value given to it by much of the public. Perhaps in our frustration with the lack of recognition, we swing the other way and promise too much.

Bragging, promising too much, and inflating the merits of our brand of work are all signs of insecurity, as is speaking negatively about other methods or practitioners. Our motivations for becoming somatic practitioners are complex, but generally, we have a desire to help people feel better. It can be difficult to tell them the simple truth—to say to someone who is in pain, for instance, "Maybe this will help, and maybe it won't. You might even feel worse before you feel better." It may be harder to say, "I don't have enough training (or skill) to help you. Let me refer you to a more advanced practitioner (or another kind of health professional)." But all professionals, no matter how advanced their skills and knowledge, need to know their limits.

THE WEEKEND WORKSHOP SYNDROME

Many of us are constantly looking for ways to advance our knowledge of ourselves and our work. We go to workshops to add new techniques to our repertoire; we attend seminars that help us with personal discovery and spiritual growth.

Weekend workshops can reenergize us and give us new ideas and techniques to explore. Personal growth workshops can free us to have healthier relationships with ourselves and our clients. But these short courses can also give fresh meaning to the phrase "A little knowledge is a dangerous thing." Sometimes weekend workshops produce "instant experts." I've seen people with a weekend workshop or two under their belts doing cervical adjustments, giving advice on neurological problems, or claiming to understand the causes of cancer. These are dangerous presumptions of expertise.

We need to feel secure in the value of our training and our work. We need to realize that the ability to give a good massage or bodywork session is as good as gold and a good somatic practitioner enhances the quality of clients' lives every day. We don't need to embellish our skills or knowledge.

We don't need to embellish our skills or knowledge. If we do what we're trained to do competently and with compassion, it's more than enough.

19

If we do what we're trained to do competently and with compassion, it's more than enough.

Some examples of what should stay outside the therapeutic circle are provided next.

MEDICAL ADVICE

Somatic practitioners' technical skills have advanced rapidly in recent years. Because of these advances, we can be confused about our role in dealing with medical situations. True, sometimes somatic practitioners have resolved physical problems that have stumped physicians, but that does not mean that we are medical experts.

> A group of bodyworkers were discussing a colleague's prospective client who had a rare disorder of the thoracic spine. Much advice was given about which vertebra to work with, which to avoid, and how to help the client. Everyone's intentions were clearly good, but all these suggestions came from practitioners who had never seen the client and knew nothing of her history or the severity of her problem. Nor did any of them have the required training to work with a client with this rare disorder.

Within the profession, there is concern about practitioners who treat medical issues without sufficient training or without consultation with the client's doctor, chiropractor, naturopath, or other involved practitioner. Such boundary violations can be as simple as giving advice that is traditionally in the medical realm such as advising a client to give up an ankle brace or to cut back on medication. Or these violations can be as dangerous as working with a client who has a serious medical condition without permission and input from the appropriate medical practitioner.

If we give an opinion, we need to identify it as a personal opinion unless it is within our scope of practice and training. And we need to take care how we state an opinion. "I've known some people who used vitamin C for colds with very good results" is safer to say than, "You should take vitamin C."

But beyond a concern for staying out of legal hot water, we want to honor the dictum, "First, do no harm." Although we can sometimes relieve a condition that wasn't helped by the usual medical regimen of drugs or surgery, that doesn't mean that we can hang out a shingle that reads, "The Doctor Is In." Most clients already give us more authority than is rightfully ours. It's up to us to stay honest and within the bounds of what we know.

PSYCHOLOGICAL COUNSELING

The hardest judgment calls to make about boundaries are those that concern psychological and emotional issues. When are we being friendly, and when are we making a mistake by acting like amateur psychotherapists? As practitioners, it's appropriate to be sensitive to our clients and supportive of them. It can be helpful to get to know them. Such information as whether

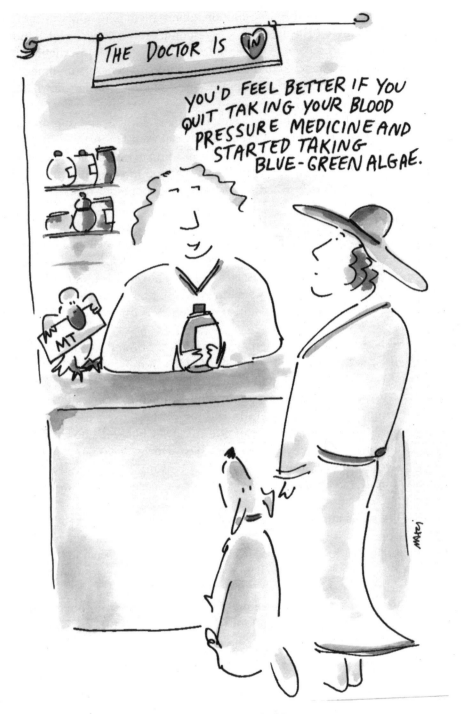

Avoid giving medical advice.

a client exercises regularly, is happily partnered, or has a stressful job can give us a broader picture of the client and help us know how to work with her better. Except for obtaining information necessary for treatment, though, it's never appropriate to pry into a client's private life.

Many clients volunteer information about their lives and concerns, making it difficult for us to know how to respond. But we have to watch that we don't stumble into the role of psychotherapist or counselor by giving advice or counseling when we don't have the training. In general, anytime our response goes beyond good listening, we're probably heading down the wrong road.

Counseling is more than just common sense. Without the appropriate education, we can't usually tell the difference between, for instance, a mentally disturbed person and someone who is reacting to a momentary or temporary crisis. We also don't usually have the training and fine tuning it takes to keep our own biases and emotional reactions out of interactions with clients.

It can be easy to fall into the trap of naively giving advice about personal matters. Our motivation is good: we want to help our clients. After all, we have our accumulated personal experience, we've read books, and maybe we've been in therapy ourselves. We may have had emotional openings that were useful or even profound. We care about our clients; we see their unhappiness and want to share our experiences and philosophies with them.

Despite their good intentions, somatic practitioners who try to act like counselors are often clumsy—doing things that a good psychotherapist would not do, such as giving advice, confronting clients bluntly, or making hasty interpretations without really knowing a client. Even if we have training in these areas, we must look at the reason the client has come to us. If he comes to us for a painful lower back, it's not our business to tell him that he's angry with his boss. However, in our role as educators, we could say, for instance, "Muscle tension is often related to our anxiety about a problem. Perhaps you've been under stress at work or at home."

On the other hand, sometimes we interpret our unspoken contract too strictly. For instance, some practitioners are uncomfortable when clients want to talk about their personal lives; they believe it isn't their job to listen to even the minor issues of a client's daily life. They want to interpret the contract very narrowly and say, "I only work with muscles."

But isn't it part of our professional role to provide an atmosphere within which clients can relax those tight muscles? Some clients unwind by talking. Although it's not our job to give advice or counseling, we can provide a sympathetic ear.

SPIRITUAL ADVICE

A client who was going through a rough time in her life complained to her new massage therapist about how difficult things were for her. The next time she saw the massage therapist, she was startled and a little put off when the therapist handed her a religious pamphlet of inspirational stories.

Regardless of how meaningful a spiritual path or religious group has been to us, it's not appropriate to set ourselves up as spiritual advisors. Sandy Fritz, author of massage therapy textbooks and a massage school director, teaches her students how to stay within boundaries with clients who seem to be dealing with bigger questions about life. She advises that when clients talk about their lives' being empty and meaningless, for instance, practitioners can help them identify that their issues might be spiritual but not give advice or deliver a sermon. Practitioners can say "Your questions strike me as involving spirituality," or "You sound as if you're thinking a lot about your fundamental beliefs about life." Such reflections may help the client clarify her quest far better than any personal advice we may be tempted to share. If we have had a spiritual experience that has been important to us, rather than being preachy, we can use that awakening to be more compassionate with our clients.

Mixing Other Businesses With Our Practice

> A massage therapist who had an outside part-time office job gave her boss a massage, not knowing that he was having marital problems with his wife, who also worked in the office. As clients sometimes do, during the massage, he began to confide in her about his unhappiness with his wife. The massage therapist felt awkward about hearing these confidences and didn't know if the boss was subtly expressing interest in her. After that encounter, she became uneasy in a work situation that had previously been comfortable.

Problems can arise from mixing business transactions—either taking on business associates as clients or trying to involve our clients in other kinds of business transactions. The former can lead, as it did in the example, to a confusion of roles, and the latter can have results that are harmful and even unethical. Suppose we sell a supplement to a client and she has an allergic reaction to it. Or, more likely, suppose we lose a client because he doesn't like feeling pressured to buy our magnets, supplements, or whatever other product we might be selling.

The most serious consideration is that it's unethical to use our relationships with clients to benefit ourselves in any way. Clients make themselves vulnerable to us and appreciate us because of the unselfish role that we take on as their practitioner. We can take advantage of that vulnerability when we try to use our influence to persuade clients to buy certain products or engage in business with us in other ways.

Boundaries Aren't Barriers

Boundaries aren't barriers between practitioner and client. Every relationship in our lives has boundaries. These limits tell us what to expect and what's appropriate in a particular situation. Boundaries are a natural part of everyone's world.

Boundaries help keep us within the limits of our training. They keep our egos and our insecurities out of our sessions, and they keep us honest. By maintaining good boundaries, we can show the best of ourselves. Good boundaries are at the heart of being a skillful and compassionate practitioner. They are what makes us professional in the eyes of the world and bring respectability and credibility to our work.

QUESTIONS FOR REFLECTION

1. Make a case for why keeping good boundaries helps clients feel safe and comfortable with us and why it matters that clients feel safe. If you don't believe that clients need to feel safe or that good boundaries help, defend that position.

2. A client tells you that she has been having an affair for the past several years with a married man who has repeatedly promised to leave his wife but has never done so. She says she doesn't know what to do and seems confused and upset. As her massage therapist, how can you respond without crossing boundaries?

3. Think back to your first professional massage. (If you haven't had a professional massage, stop right now and go get one.) Were you nervous? Did you know what to expect? Is there anything that the practitioner could have told you either on the phone or when you first arrived that could have made you more comfortable or that would have helped you know what to expect?

4. Has a professional of any kind ever given you advice that was outside his or her level of expertise and also unasked-for? How did you feel about that?

5. Your office has just been blown away by a tornado. As you stand in the rubble that was once your treatment room, your 4:00 client arrives. What can you say to the client that would be client-centered?

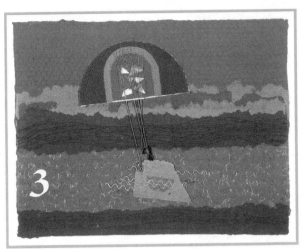

Chapter 3

*F*RAMEWORK: NUTS AND BOLTS OF BOUNDARIES

Framework issues can sound dry and dull. Who wants to talk about the joy of starting sessions on time and the delights of clean sheets? But it is in those details that we define our practices as professional. As discussed in previous chapters, our clients are vulnerable; they need good boundaries in order to trust us. Framework details are the nuts and bolts of good boundaries.

Many somatic practitioners' careers have suffered because of carelessness about the details that make clients comfortable. Clients care about those issues more than we may be aware.

Here's an eye-opening conversation I had with a friend:

> I asked my old friend Robbie what made her a loyal client of her massage therapist. "She's very competent," she said. Since Robbie is an art history professor and doesn't know effleurage from petrissage, I was curious how she came to that conclusion. She thought for a minute and said, "Her tapes are long enough."
>
> She meant that the massage therapist was careful to have music that lasted for the whole session, so she didn't have to fumble around with changing tapes and interrupt the flow. She added that the room is always clean and tidy, the table is heated, and the therapist doesn't talk unless Robbie initiates a conversation. Also, Robbie felt the therapist never gives a massage-by-the-numbers but always homes in on where Robbie's aches and pains are that week.

Our clients know little about the technical part of our work. Our offices are foreign territory to them. The only way they can judge our competence and caring is by our professional behavior and whether they feel safe with us.

Framework: The logistics by which we define ourselves as professional and create a safe atmosphere for our clients. Framework includes the ways that we present ourselves in advertising, the preparation of the physical setting, our policies on fees and time, and such ground rules as keeping the focus on the client.

Framework details are the nuts and bolts of good boundaries.

The ability to create an atmosphere within which clients can make use of our work is crucial. We may rush to learn the latest techniques and pride ourselves on our sensitivity, but our effectiveness may depend on whether or not, in a manner of speaking, our tapes are long enough.

The Need for Framework: Holding the Space

Some practitioners call it "holding the space." Others call it "creating a container." They recognize that clients need to have a special environment that is focused solely on their well-being. Attending to framework is more than simply buying massage oil and soothing music; we need to take care of all the details that make us professional. Careless framework can interfere with the therapeutic process. A colleague reports:

> I used to be a massage therapist in a holistic center in which no one had an assigned office. Instead, we used whatever room was available at the time. Sometimes my client and I had to wait 10 or 15 minutes until a room was free. We rarely worked in the same room two times in a row. The other practitioners and I often talked about how uptight our clients seemed to be. Now I see that their difficulty letting go was probably a response to our erratic setup. How could they relax in such an unstable environment?

When the framework isn't stable, sometimes clients are uncomfortable without knowing why. They just feel out of sorts. They may be more demanding or more tense than they would be if they felt safe and attended to. Practitioners also are affected by unreliable framework. Not only are we more likely to be dealing with cranky clients, but also we can be drained by the lack of stability in our work lives.

There *are* good practitioners who are careless with framework yet seem to have healthy practices. Clients sometimes forgive other omissions if the practitioner has a terrific personality or great technical skills. Yet even in those cases, clients notice and respond positively if those practitioners start attending to framework issues. And the practitioners find they have fewer "difficult" clients and more energy at the end of the day.

> A popular massage therapist worked for years out of a room in her home that was less than neat—in fact, it was a cluttered mess. Despite that, she was successful because she was a good listener and a sensitive bodyworker, plus she was professional in every other way.
> Recently, she complained that her work seemed to take more and more energy over the years. I suggested that she try simply tidying up the room. I thought that she wouldn't have to work as hard to create a professional atmosphere if the room said it for her. It was a small change, but she reported that cleaning up the room made a difference. She looks forward to her work more in this neater, more professional office and reports that new clients seem to settle in and relax faster.

Some practitioners have great personalities or amazing skills. For the rest of us, the majority, who are charismatically impaired and less-than-dazzling technicians, attention to framework balances our shortcomings. Consistency, care for the client, and the ability to set limits well can go a long way toward a solid, satisfying practice. And we will last longer in this profession.

Framework Basics: Setting the Stage

Our work with clients begins long before they walk through the door. It starts with the first phone call or even the first time they see our business card. We need to take care of how we present ourselves from the very beginning. With every detail of setting up a practice, we need to consider the basics of the professional therapeutic relationship. For instance, any advertising—whether it's putting up a business card at the health food store, running an ad in the newspaper, or creating a website—should involve clear and honest information about who we are and what we do. Ads are the beginning of educating clients about what to expect from us.

Business Cards

Business cards usually won't make or break a practice. Some practitioners with successful practices have unimpressive-looking cards. However, your card is one more piece of information about you; you want it to give clients a favorable impression and perhaps a sense of your personal style.

Business cards should be simple and eye catching. Avoid making a long list of the techniques and modalities you offer, especially if they are techniques that are unfamiliar to most of the public. Some cards look like a smorgasbord: "Mary Smith—Hypnotherapy, Past Life Regression, Acupressure, Sports Massage, and Palm Reading." That hodgepodge of services can be bewildering to the public, and prospective clients could also be skeptical that, unless Mary Smith is 103 years old, she can't be really good at all of those things.

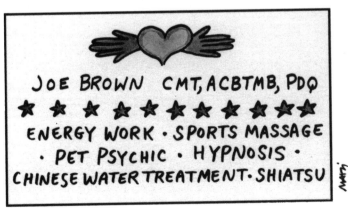

Long lists on business cards can be confusing.

Beware of using only your first name on a business card. It may look as though you have a reason to hide your identity, and it's also the way that sex workers advertise in the newspaper. Not a good idea. You might also think twice about using cute names, such as "We Knead U." The tone is friendly and humorous but could be seen as making a joke of your work.

Having a business card shows people that you're serious about your work; people expect professionals to have business cards. Also, the process of designing a card often helps you clarify what tone you want to set for your business and what you want people to know about you.

Advertising and Reaching the Public

Where and how to advertise varies depending on where you live. It may sound obvious, but first decide what population you want to reach and then figure out how to contact them. It's a good idea to talk with colleagues and more experienced practitioners in your area to see what has worked for them. As with business cards, advertising needs to be simple and attractive. Massage is such a personal service that you may not receive many calls from impersonal advertising alone, but it does help prospective clients to begin to associate your name with your business.

Speaking to groups about massage is one good way to advertise. Once people have met you (assuming you appear friendly and professional), they are more likely to feel comfortable making an appointment. Such presentations can include a short talk on the benefits of massage or your particular kind of massage, followed by a brief demonstration. The demonstration can be, for instance, a foot massage on a clothed volunteer. It helps if people can see the care and concern with which you approach your clients. Your talk can include enough technical detail or anatomical references to show people that you know what you are doing; however, keep in mind that most people just want to know if you can help them feel better.

Websites

A website is a useful piece of advertising: unlike business cards and ads, websites give you room to explain your kind of bodywork, beliefs, credentials, fees, and answers to typical concerns. You can put your website's address on your business card and give prospective clients the opportunity to find out more about you. A website doesn't need to be elaborate and large—just attractive, professional, and informative. It's another way to convey your own style and values. As with any advertising, it's a good idea to get feedback from colleagues and mentors before making it official.

Phone and Voice Mail Guidelines

What prospective clients hear when they first call your business phone number is an important part of setting the stage. Very few somatic practitioners have an office with a receptionist. Most have various ways—such as beepers, voice mail, and answering machines—for people to contact them and leave messages. No matter what your preference, you want to be easily accessible, sound professional, and provide privacy for your clients and prospective clients. This is often the first contact the public has with you, and you don't want it to be the last.

Right from the start you can demonstrate the elements of the professional relationship. For instance, to be client-centered in your first contact, put yourself in the client's position. What kind of message would you want to hear if you were calling a stranger to ask her or him to work with you in a highly personal way?

Other boundaries come into play here. For clients' confidentiality, you need to have a way that they can leave a message that only you can access. If your phone line is shared with colleagues, family members, or others, it is fairly inexpensive and easy to add a separate box to your answering system and a message of "Press 1 for Susie." Alternately, a voice mail service or cell phone exclusively for your business is a good choice. These options also avoid the boundary problem of giving clients an unnecessary glimpse into your private life. Even if you live in a small town and everyone knows a good deal about your personal life, prospective clients will be comforted to know that you keep your business separate and guard your clients' privacy.

For clients' confidentiality, you need to have a way that they can leave a message that only you can access.

It's unprofessional and violates confidentiality to allow client's messages to be heard by your family members or anyone other than staff members who are trained to keep confidentiality. Even the fact that someone is a client should be kept private. A colleague reports:

> I once worked with a small group of therapists and bodyworkers in a situation where everyone shared a phone line, and each of us could hear the others' messages as they looked for their own. More than once, I heard parts of private messages from people that I knew (and sometimes didn't know were in therapy with one of the counselors) that I'm sure the person wouldn't have wanted me to hear. Just the sound of a client's voice when that person is feeling needy is too personal for your colleague, partner, or family member to hear.

Your phone greetings should be warm but businesslike and to the point. There's no need to be clever and say something like, "This is John's answering machine." Everyone knows by now that a machine isn't really talking on its own. And does anyone really enjoy having to listen to a musical prelude when they reach someone's answering machine? Prospective clients usually appreciate a short, relevant, friendly message.

If you take and return business calls from your home, make sure the television isn't blaring in the background and your children aren't being noisy. For incoming calls, use a screening device such as caller ID so you can choose when to answer. Allowing friends and family members to answer your business calls can lead to problems. For instance, a boyfriend answering the phone may send out more information about your life than the client needs. And a small child answering the phone might be endearing but also might be annoying. Even one minute of repeating, "Is your mommy home?" may give new clients second thoughts about making an appointment with a new practitioner. They may wonder if the practitioner's family life will interfere with her professional life in other ways.

The First Phone Conversation

The therapeutic relationship starts with the first conversation.

The therapeutic relationship starts with the first conversation. Rob Bauer, Rubenfeld synergist, notes, "Complex dynamics are already in process during the first phone call. Clients are imagining things, intuiting things, and noticing things about you—whether you live with someone, how excited you are about your work, or whether you're sensitive."

Be informative and reassuring, but don't sound as if you're reading from a set speech. Know how you want to answer the usual questions: your fees, your hours, and the particular benefits of your modality. (Chapter 8 gives tips about how to deal with clients looking for sexual services as well as with advertising to avoid such misunderstandings.) Because commonly asked questions may vary depending on the modality or even what region of the country you live in, it's a good idea for new practitioners to ask more experienced colleagues in their area for advice about this first phone call. Also, you don't want to stumble around when prospective clients ask you the benefits of your work. Rehearse with a friend.

Much can be learned about clients in the initial phone call. Do they, for instance, want to share a great deal of personal information or ask for advice? You can start setting boundaries in that first call by letting them know that some issues are best dealt with during office visits. Be careful about letting people take up an unusual amount of time on the phone; it sets a bad precedent. Even with these earliest contacts, it's important to be aware of setting limits to protect yourself.

If a client asks for an appointment tomorrow at 3:00 and you don't have that opening, you don't need to apologize and ramble on, as if to a friend, about why you can't see them then. Clients simply want to know what appointment you *do* have open

The first phone call is a great opportunity to educate the client. You can set the stage for the session:

> Arnold Katz, a massage therapist in Boston, says that, even in the first phone call, after a client has made an appointment, he explains what will happen in the session very thoroughly so there's no mystery. He takes clients through the session step by step from the minute they come in the door—that he will take a physical history, that he will then leave the room so that they can get undressed, that they will lie under a sheet and be draped at all times, and so forth. He lets them know from the beginning that if they are uncomfortable in any way, at any time, he wants them to speak up right away.

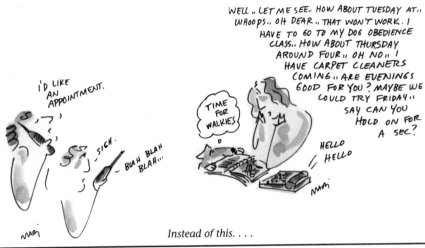

Instead of this. . . .

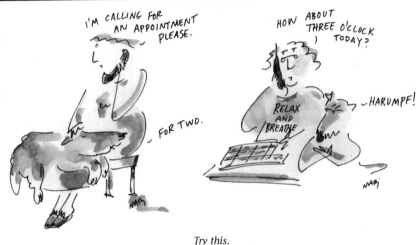

Try this.

Aside from honoring clients' right to informed consent, letting new clients know what to expect can help them be more at ease when they arrive for their first session.

Framework Basics: The Setting

A therapy room that feels safe and inviting to clients will benefit your practice and be a joy for you to work in.

Home or Office?

Where to locate your practice is a personal choice that depends on a number of factors, including cost and convenience. If you can afford it, working out of an office rather than a home is generally more professional and will feel safer both to you and to your clients. A client reports:

When I first started getting bodywork, I made an appointment with a male practitioner I didn't know. Even though he'd been well recommended, I was uncomfortable because he worked out of his house. When I went for that first appointment, I actually gave a friend the practitioner's address and said, "If I don't call you in 2 hours, call the police." The session went fine, but I want bodyworkers to know that their business can be affected if they work out of their homes.

Separating Work Space and Personal Life

The more you separate your work and your personal life, the better. If you choose to work out of your home, use a room that's set aside just for your professional work. The message to clients is that this is a space solely for clients. There's also an advantage to being able to shut the office door at the end of your business day and focus on your private life without reminders of work concerns.

When working out of your home, the best arrangement is to have a separate entrance for clients or a way for them to access your office without getting a view of your private living space. Having a separate bathroom for clients is also ideal.

Whether your office is in your home or outside it, you want it to feel warm and inviting to your clients but still professional and not overwhelmingly personal. If you work out of your home, you don't want your office space to look like a bedroom with a massage table in it—eliminate bedroom-type furniture and large numbers of personal pictures and items. There's no harm in having a couple of family pictures in the room—in fact, it can be reassuring to clients to see that a practitioner is married or has children. Also, a picture of the practitioner's partner or spouse may discourage a client from making romantic overtures.

Practitioners need to avoid making their offices into displays of their personal beliefs—political, spiritual, or otherwise. Clients may feel excluded if they don't share your beliefs, or they may have judgments about your beliefs that will affect how they feel about you.

Preparing the Room

Clients love coming into a room that's all set up for them—neat, warm sheets on the table and everything ready to go. Ready rooms are an immediate sign of your professionalism and caring.

Clients won't feel comfortable in unclean rooms or surroundings. Clients don't find it charming when the cat jumps on their bare back with sticky kitty-littered feet (true story) or when the room is obviously dirty or the bathroom is a mess. With so many new viruses and bacteria popping up these days, people are concerned about catching something. Find a balance between a room that smells antiseptic and one that feels as though germs may be lurking in every corner. (Also, remember to wash your hands before and after you work with a client. Although that sounds obvious, if doctors forget to do it—and studies show that they do—manual therapists probably do, too.) The need for order and cleanliness in the environment can go deeper for some clients. After all, some people grow up with ideas about their bodies being "dirty" and may feel a heightened sensitivity when they come for bodywork. Clean, orderly surroundings help clients relax.

There's a saying, "Heaven is in the details." Professionalism calls for a heavenly attention to the finer aspects of how you present yourself and your work and how you welcome clients into your practice.

Draping

Appropriate draping of clients is required for privacy and comfort. If a client asks not to be draped, advise the client that it's part of your professional standards that every client be draped. There's no really good reason to allow a client not to be draped. The manual therapy profession is still striving to separate its public image from that of sex workers, and appropriate draping is a simple, easy way you can define that difference.

Basic Session Framework

Erratic framework affects both client and practitioner. Clients may feel nervous or fussy in a confused framework, and practitioners may respond by being harried or drained by the end of the day. For instance, imagine being careless with just one aspect of framework, such as starting and ending on time. How would you feel if you ran late all day? Imagine how it would feel to be the client of someone who was never on time.

The following framework guidelines provide a solid structure for your work. If these guidelines sound too much like rules, try thinking of them as small acts of kindness toward vulnerable clients. They are also small acts of self-discipline that will make your work life run more smoothly. If you aren't already using these guidelines, you may want to try them out and see if you notice a positive difference. (Practitioners who have been scattered about framework in the past will need to be consistently careful for some time before noticing a difference.)

Session Framework Guidelines:[1]

- Clients know what to expect and what is expected of them.
- Sessions start and end on time.
- Sessions occur at the same time and place at regular intervals.
- Nothing interrupts a session.
- Practitioners avoid casual discussion of treatment or sessions with clients outside office boundaries.

[1]Adapted from Narboe N. Working With What You Can't Get Your Hands On. Portland, OR: Narboe, 1985.

- Practitioners carefully safeguard clients' rights to privacy and confidentiality.
- Clients are unaware of each other.
- Practitioners don't ask clients to attend to their needs.

Clients Know What to Expect and What Is Expected of Them

Before you begin the hands-on work, you need to receive the informed consent of the client. You can ask the client to sign a consent form that explains your credentials, the nature of the treatment, and the possible benefits and side effects. Advise the client in written or verbal form about any consequences of the treatment such as muscle soreness or lightheadedness. Assure clients that they have the right to refuse any procedure at any time. Clients should also be advised during the session when you want to introduce any treatment procedure not previously agreed to and when you are going to be working near the breasts, anus, or genitals.

The agreement the client signs should also give details about fees and cancellation policies and any other financial policies, such as procedures for bad checks.

Procedures regarding confidentiality should be part of the initial intake and are discussed later in the section on confidentiality.

Sessions Start and End on Time

Time boundaries help make a safe container—they define the professional situation as different from a social one and put limits on the nature of the relationship. Starting on time is respectful of both your time and the client's. For instance, if a client shows up early for an appointment, you still want to start the session at the appointed time. Don't let a client cut into the time you've set aside to rest or return messages. If a client with a 3:00 appointment arrives at 2:45, you can greet her with a smile and say, "I see you're early. Just have a seat in the waiting area. I'll be ready for you at 3:00."

Ending on time is just as important. "If you don't end your session on time, your client will never trust you," says Sandra Wooten, director of Rosen Method Center Southwest. Clients like to know what to expect and schedule other parts of their lives based on those expectations. Unpredictable practitioners can make clients uneasy. If you go long one session because the client is in pain, she may think you'll go short next time if she's not and may begin to come up with a new pain at the end of each session.

Being consistent about time has many advantages for practitioners. If you're usually consistent but find yourself always wanting to go over or under the usual amount of time with a certain client, that can be a sign that you need to look at why you are treating that client differently. It also makes it easier to monitor yourself in other ways. If you want to take extra time with *every* client, you may be trying too hard, and if you want to cut the session short with every client, you may be approaching burnout.

Even if clients are still experiencing intense emotion or pain, ending close to the agreed-on time can provide comforting structure. Lengthening sessions a great deal because there is still pain or emotion could tell clients that you think you are responsible for their pain rather than that your job is to do your best within a certain time limit. It may also show that you don't trust that the work you've already done will have results or that your clients have other resources as well.

If you have any clients who have a pattern of requesting additional work at the end of a session, it might be a good idea to inform them how much time is left, perhaps about 10 minutes before the end of the session, and ask if they have any areas that need special attention during the remaining time.

What "ending on time" means varies from practitioner to practitioner. Many somatic practitioners don't schedule precisely on the hour or half hour; they allow for a little extra work time on the table, gathering-up time for slow-moving clients, or breathing room for themselves. The amount of time varies from practitioner to practitioner, but 15 minutes is usually enough leeway. Those who are doing emotionally oriented bodywork, such as practitioners of the Rosen Method or the Rubenfeld Synergy Method, are careful to end after an hour because more precise boundaries are needed for work that deals with deep emotional issues.

Being consistent about time doesn't mean that you need to be rigid; sometimes a client is in an unusual crisis. A massage therapist told of taking an extra 30 minutes with a client whose mother had just died. (The therapist wasn't disrupting other clients' schedules by doing so.) A bodyworker said she scheduled extra time with a client who had come a long distance to work with her.

It's also a good idea, even if your practice isn't full, to schedule and end sessions on time as if you were solidly booked. It's good discipline, and it shows clients that you value your time. Your practice will run much more smoothly, and your clients will be more secure.

Sessions Occur at the Same Time and Place at Regular Intervals

Although you're not in control of whether your clients come back regularly, be aware of the importance of consistency and try to keep clients in the same time slot. If you have to bounce a client out of a regular time or if you're relocating your practice to a different office, you want to be aware of keeping the other parts of the framework on an even keel. Moves and changes can upset clients without their fully realizing it.

When you do have to see clients at a time other than their usual one or when you move to a new office, you may notice that clients behave differently—they may be pickier, more off balance, more insecure in some way. You may have to make an extra effort to help them feel comfortable. You could make a comment to show them that you understand how unsettling such an adjustment can be. For instance, if they're acting rattled, you could say, "It must feel strange to come in at a different time (or be in a new office)."

Nothing Interrupts a Session

All of these guidelines are based on the central idea that being professional means that the focus is on the client. Clients are paying for your time and attention. You don't want your pager going off, the doorbell ringing, or any other kind of interruption. There are very few good reasons to answer the phone during a session. (Perhaps if you knew that the Nobel Peace Prize committee was going to call during that hour . . . but even so, you would need to warn the client of a possible interruption.) Make sure you have turned off all your phones and pagers (and whatever other communication devices modern technology comes up with) and ask your clients to do so as well. Some clients will balk at that, but you can at least make a strong suggestion, letting them know how counterproductive it can be for their cell phone to ring when they are deeply relaxed.

Practitioners who work at home need to keep the environment as free of interruptions as possible—for example, put a "Do Not Disturb" sign on the front door and advise friends not to drop by and family members not to interfere.

If an interruption is unavoidable (the sink is stopped up, and the plumber is coming), let clients know before the session starts that there may be a brief interruption and that you will make up the time lost. If you know before the appointment time that a session may be interrupted, you can even call clients and forewarn them.

Practitioners should do their utmost to see that no one walks in on a session. Clients will be startled by that, no matter who the intruder is. A friend relates:

> One of my most uncomfortable massages was from a woman who worked out of her living room and had a 3-year-old child. Throughout the massage, whenever I opened my eyes, I'd see the curious little girl peeking in. She didn't say anything or actively take her mother's attention, but just having her there took away my privacy.

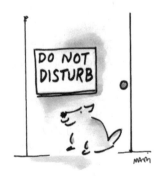

Practitioners Avoid Casual Discussion of Treatment or Sessions With Clients Outside Office Boundaries

It's a boundary violation to initiate casual conversation with a client about his treatment outside a session. When you see clients in another setting, you may be tempted to talk about their last session: "Is your back still sore?" or "I hope you're feeling better." These may seem like innocent remarks, but when you carry your therapeutic role to another setting, you confuse the boundaries. The safety of your office setting allows clients to relax and show sides of themselves that they might not ordinarily show, both physically and emotionally. Aside from showing their unclothed bodies, they may, for instance, show a more dependent or needy aspect of themselves that isn't usually part of the face they present to the public. When you see clients at the grocery store and say cheerfully, "Hi, how's your back?", you've just, in effect, dragged their naked and vulnerable body into the store.

When clients see you outside the office and initiate a conversation about the last session or their physical symptoms, it is a great time to practice setting limits. "You broke your toe? Oh my goodness, that's too bad. Give me a call, and let's set up a time when I can see you." Or, as you back slowly away smiling, "Oh, how interesting. We can talk about that next time you come in."

Of course, if clients contact you by phone or e-mail and have questions or concerns about previous sessions or their responses to them, you need to answer their questions and address their concerns. You want to set aside time in your workday to respond to such calls. However, you should avoid talking with clients about treatment concerns at public places or social gatherings or any time or place outside your office or outside the time you have set aside to answer or receive business calls.

The Internet has opened up new areas for boundary complications. Some Internet providers have "instant messaging" features that enable customers to know when another customer is online and then "chat" with him. Despite the seeming anonymity of socializing online, Internet boundaries should follow the same guidelines as in-person boundaries. Avoid exchanging anything but minimal social greetings with clients outside the office, even if the connection is electronic. You also want to be careful about giving clients your e-mail address.

Practitioners Carefully Safeguard Clients' Rights to Privacy and Confidentiality

Nothing that goes on in your sessions—either what clients say or their physical situation or reactions—should be conveyed to others. You shouldn't give others information about a client without the client's (usually written) permission, nor should you repeat anything a client says in a session, no matter how seemingly insignificant. Even the fact that someone is a client should be kept private. (Situations in which you can make exceptions to confidentiality rules are discussed in Chapter 5.)

The Health Insurance Portability and Accountability Act (HIPAA) sets forth strict confidentiality guidelines that apply to practitioners who use electronic means (faxes and computers) to send information about clients to insurers for billing purposes or who obtain information about clients from medical practitioners.[2]

It is beyond the scope of this book to discuss these guidelines in detail, and practitioners to whom the HIPAA requirements apply should seek more complete guidelines.[3] However, all practitioners need to be aware of procedures for obtaining permission and guarding privacy.

OBTAINING PERMISSION

During the intake process, along with getting the client's consent for treatment, you should have the client sign a permission form that enables you to obtain information about the client from other health care practitioners and give information about the client to other health care practitioners, as needed. If you plan to discuss your clients in supervision or consultation, you should also have written permission from the client to do so. Keep in mind that the client has the right to refuse to give permission. You should also give clients a written statement of your privacy and confidentiality policies, letting them know that you will safeguard all information about them.

For reasons of their privacy, you must have clients' permission to call or write them at their home or office. Let them know that on some occasions you may need to cancel or change an appointment and ask them how they would like to be contacted. If you are trying to reach a client and must leave a message with someone other than the client or on a shared answering machine, do not identify yourself as that person's massage therapist (or polarity therapist, Alexander teacher, and so on.)

If you send marketing pieces or special offers in the mail, it's best to get written permission from your clients to send them material. Use a form that the client can sign for all of these permissions so that you can keep a clear record of them.

GUARDING PRIVACY

It's important that no one else has access to information about your clients without your consent. Keep all information about clients in a locked file or some place that others cannot get into, and keep your appointment book and clients' checks out of public view. Staff members such as receptionists also need to know how to keep clients information private.

Respecting confidentiality also means that arrangements should be made so that people walking by your office door can't overhear the talk during a session. An easy way to block sound is to use a machine that makes white noise. You can also use a solid door, a double door, or a door with soundproofing at the bottom and top. Double doors—adding another door

---

[2]http://www.hipaa.org/
[3]Sohnen-Moe C. An Update on HIPAA. Massage & Bodywork, December/January 2004.

that hinges on the other side from the one already there—are also helpful for privacy. In a busy office, they give you a way to come and go without accidentally giving someone in the hall a glimpse of the client.

Clients Are Unaware of Each Other

Some therapists who do classic psychotherapy or psychoanalysis arrange their schedules and office entrances and exits so that clients don't see each other. One client leaves from one door at 10 minutes to the hour, and the next one comes in a different door on the hour. The goal is to maintain clients' privacy and cut down on the potential for their imaginings about the therapist's relationship with other clients.

I don't know any somatic practitioners (and few psychotherapists) who separate clients' entrances and exits. Most don't even think to schedule clients so that they arrive and leave without seeing each other. But it's a good idea. You don't know how it will affect one client to see you being warm and friendly as you say good-bye to the previous client at the door; it may mean nothing, but it may stir up the client's insecurity.

A colleague reports:

> Waiting to get a session from a much-loved bodywork teacher, I saw him walk out of his previous session with his arm around his client, chatting in a friendly way. I felt great annoyance and dismay and watched myself spin off into a negative internal monologue: "He doesn't do that with me. He likes that other client better than he likes me. He probably doesn't like me at all."

Because my colleague had a solid history of trusting that teacher, her reaction didn't last and the situation didn't interfere with the session, but it could have been disruptive. It could have been one of those sessions when the practitioner didn't understand why the client was being "difficult."

Arranging for clients to leave without bumping into someone else is also considerate of the fact that, as they leave your office, they're not always in a frame of mind to deal with other people. They may think their hair looks messy, or they may be tearful or not in a state to want to make polite chitchat.

The goal is for clients to be unaware of your professional relationships with other clients. For this reason (and for confidentiality), you don't name your clients to each other. Even if you don't say another client's name but give information about her, it gives the impression that you are loose with clients' privacy, and it takes the focus off the present client. Occasionally, it might be reassuring to a client to hear that others have the same kinds of problems. For instance, you could say, "I've noticed that many of my clients seem tenser during the holidays." However, in deciding whether to make such a comment, you should be motivated by what is best for the client.

Create a setting in which each client knows that he or she is the most important person in your (work) life for that hour. There's probably not a client in the world who is interested in seeing his practitioner warmly embrace another client or hearing him talk about another client. Why run the risk of stirring up something that will interfere with the client's trust?

Practitioners Don't Ask Clients to Attend to Their Needs

It's never appropriate to ask clients to take care of you—even in the smallest way.

It's never appropriate to ask clients to take care of you—even in the smallest way. A practitioner might be tempted to ask for such care in an obvious way, such as trying to get sympathy about a difficult divorce or asking for advice about a client's area of expertise. Also, practitioners with good intentions may have the misguided idea that it's friendly or somehow helpful to clients to be open with them about personal issues. Actually, it can be a distraction in what is *their* time. What is truly helpful to clients is giving them your full attention, not bringing your personal life into the session, and not asking paying customers to give out emotional support or free advice.

There are subtle ways you could ask clients to take care of your needs. You might say things such as, "Boy, I've had a rough day," "I don't like this hot weather," or "I was up so late last night." Even these subtle messages can create problems. Maybe you've had a hard day, but so have they—they're counting on you to help their day be easier. When they hear something that sounds like you're not up to snuff that day, it can interfere with their ability to let go and focus on their own experience, and they may fear they're not going to get their money's worth.

Clients are paying you to put aside your personal needs and do what's best for them. Personal revelations from the practitioner can be off-putting. They may begin to see you, in small ways, as needy and inadequate to handle their problems. They may also get the mistaken idea that you want to have a personal relationship with them.

You're not being deceptive when you keep your personal needs out of sessions; it's just good professional manners. You're not arrogantly pretending that you don't have needs; you're simply being appropriate to the professional setting.

Framework With Clients at Different Stages

When is framework important? Although clients may be at different stages in their relationships with us or have particular needs, the importance of framework doesn't change. As these examples suggest, framework is important to all of our clients.

New Clients

The first appointment is crucial for setting a professional tone. Clients put off by sloppy framework in the first session simply don't come back. There are no second chances. With a regular client, if you are late, have a messy office, or make an inappropriate comment, the client will probably dismiss it as a momentary lapse. But with a new client who can only judge you by that one appointment, such carelessness can imply indifference or incompetence.

Regular Clients

Regular clients get used to their routines, and their hour may feel like a safe haven. Avoid taking clients out of their patterns. If you have to change the framework—move offices or raise fees, for example—be sensitive in presenting those changes. You need to give clients ample notice (a month or two) about major changes.

Clients of Structural Bodywork or Deep Emotional Work

In deep structural bodywork, when clients' physical (and emotional) patterns are shifting, they need a stable therapeutic environment. The same holds true for psychologically or emotionally oriented bodywork. The more you expect the client to access deep emotional material, the more care you need to take with framework.

Mentally Disturbed Clients

If you're working with clients whose internal process is chaotic, you need to be more attentive to external boundaries. This can be difficult because these clients' own sense of boundaries is usually so scattered that they tend not to honor yours. They may want special exceptions, as in this case:

> A colleague working with a mentally unbalanced woman reported that his limit-setting abilities were challenged when the client requested that he lower her fee, give her a ride to the session, and work only with one specific area, even though the practitioner's methods called for a whole-body approach.

Some mentally unbalanced clients will be outside the scope of your abilities as a bodyworker, and you will need advice from a mental health professional to make an appropriate referral. However, with others, gentle firmness and consistency are enough to settle them down.

Clients Who Are Traumatized or in Pain

Fear and pain make us more sensitive to orderliness and kindness in the environment. Clients who have experienced a good deal of trauma in their lives may be vigilant and watchful, expecting danger at every moment. Clients frightened by chronic physical pain are like wounded animals that have retreated into a corner. Both kinds of clients can be hypersensitive to any perceived imbalance in the therapeutic relationship. Small framework errors or lapses in attention can make them think we are incompetent or indifferent. Such clients are grateful for good boundaries.

Clients With Whom You Have Another Relationship

You can be tempted to be careless about framework with people you know: "I don't have to have the room ready—it's only my buddy Bob." You actually need to be *more* crisp with your boundaries in such cases to help friends with the confusion of switching roles.

Clients Who Have Been Sexually Abused

Extra attention to framework is necessary for clients who have been sexually abused. At the same time, because their own boundaries may be confused, they may push the edges—being flirtatious with you or asking for special treatment. To keep your boundaries safe enough for these clients, part of your framework should include supervision from a mental health professional.

Ending the Professional Relationship: Achieving Closure

You want to do your best to end your professional relationship with clients on a positive note. Leaving clients with negative feelings could color how they evaluate their entire time working with you or leave them with bad feelings about the profession in general.

Contacting Clients Who Quit

Sometimes when regular clients suddenly stop making appointments without giving a reason, you may wonder whether to contact them. You may be concerned that you have somehow offended them or made them uncomfortable. Generally, when clients stop coming and you have decided to contact them, it's a good idea to write a note (handwritten, not e-mailed) and say that you've noticed their absence and that you hope they're doing well. If you have reason to believe you've offended them, you can say that you hope that you haven't inadvertently offended or upset them and that you're open to talking about any concerns they might have. A note is less confrontational than a phone call and easier for both practitioner and client to handle.

When a regular client stops seeing you abruptly, your decision about what to do may be influenced by your personal feelings. You may, for instance, feel angry, rejected, or just plain disappointed. If you're confused about what to do or say or if you have many feelings about this client's leaving, it would be a good time to talk with a trusted teacher or colleague in a confidential setting to help sort out your feelings. You might even consult with a professional who is knowledgeable about interpersonal dynamics—such as a counselor, psychotherapist, or bodyworker who has psychological training—to help you clarify your response to the situation. (Such a consultation wouldn't involve delving into personal issues as you would in psychotherapy. It would only help you with smoothing out issues that get in the way of good relationships with clients.)

Moving Out of Town and Ending Your Practice

If even small changes in framework are disruptive to clients, what is it like for them when you leave town or end your practice? If you terminate with clients carelessly, you may leave them with a bad feeling about the whole experience of working with you.

You want to give clients adequate notice so that they can get used to the idea of their sessions ending and have time to express their feelings, whether those feelings are anger, rejection, gratitude, or some combination. If you are able, 2 months is a good amount of time to give notice. You can send notes to clients who don't come in regularly so that they don't have a rude surprise when they call for an appointment. Also, be prepared with names of other practitioners to whom you can refer them.

For practitioners, too, it's often emotionally difficult to leave; you may be grieving the loss created by the change or feeling guilty, as if you were abandoning your clients. During this time, getting support from trusted teachers or a professional trained in psychological dynamics can help make the transition smoother so that you can more effectively help clients—and yourself—weather the change.

Bending Framework: A Red Flag

A good reason for being consistent with boundaries is that you will be more inclined to notice when you alter them. It's a red flag when you step outside your usual framework. When you bend your professional boundaries, you encourage others to treat you as if you're not a professional. When boundaries become like Swiss cheese, clients can fall through the holes.

Les Kertay, clinical psychologist and former chair of the Rolf Institute's ethics committee, says that making special exceptions for clients is always a red flag for practitioners. One of the main ways people get into big trouble with clients (ethics complaints, for instance) or even small trouble (the client doesn't come back or becomes a "difficult" client) is through treating the client as "special" in some way.

A colleague relates:

> There has been only one time in my 20 years of practice when I didn't get paid—and it was a client for whom I had made exception after exception. I allowed my judgment to be clouded for a number of reasons: she had a large area of scar tissue on her chest and neck from a traumatic childhood injury, she said she was in a great deal of pain, and she was a struggling single mother.
>
> Rushing in to rescue her, I discounted my fee substantially and would see her at times when I didn't usually schedule sessions. She never seemed to get relief from the pain, and that would double my desire to fix her. The last time I saw her, I agreed to work on my birthday, although I had planned to take the day off. To make it worse, I was giving her a discount. At the end of the session, she said she didn't have any checks with her and that she would mail me the fee. That was the last I heard from her. Stiffed on my birthday—it's a lesson I remember. I had created a framework disaster.

Would it have been hard hearted not to make an exception for a client in great pain? You want to distinguish between a client who is sincerely in a crisis and a client who has a pattern of being manipulative. That can be a difficult judgment call, but there are often clues. For example, a client may call and say that she is in terrible distress and must be seen right away. If the practitioner says, for instance, "I can't see you Sunday, but I have an opening at 10 a.m. on Monday," and the client responds, "Oh, I can't then. That's when I get my hair cut", or provides another seemingly flimsy excuse, the client isn't being straightforward. Other clients may describe awful pain and want to be seen immediately, but when the practitioner asks how long they've had the pain, they'll say, "Six years." Their pain may be real, but you may not need to rearrange your schedule to see them right away.

You don't do clients a favor when you let them hook you into ignoring your own framework policies. You also don't need to judge clients who want to be treated in a special way. The client who didn't pay was simply dealing with a difficult situation in an unhealthy way that she'd learned a long time ago. It was a mistake for the practitioner to continue to treat her in a special way, and it wasn't helpful to the client. People heal best when they have a safe container, and this client never knew where the boundaries were.

If someone has been injured or is in emotional crisis, depending on the circumstances and your schedule, you may want to make an exception for him or her. Special exceptions need to be carefully considered and consistent. Experienced practitioners develop their own guidelines about what circumstances will warrant bending the standard framework, and they then avoid going outside their own rules. Firm framework saves energy and stress and provides comfort for both practitioner and client.

Framework Matters

What individual clients need in order to feel safe varies. There are guidelines, such as confidentiality, that are universally part of a professional code. Others may lend themselves to flexibility. For instance, in some cases, because of either the practitioner's personality or the client's, a cluttered treatment room may not make a difference. In other cases, messiness could make a client uncomfortable. The ultimate authority for framework is the client's experience. Does what you do make your clients tense or help them breathe easier?

Maintaining a stable framework also benefits you. An inconsistent framework—variations in how long sessions run, special deals with fees, for instance—is energy consuming for practitioners.

Although you want to be consistent and stable in your framework, experienced practitioners know that total consistency is an ideal rather than a reality. The point is not to become rigidly locked into rules but to know that framework matters and to thoughtfully consider the ways you manage the nuts and bolts of your practice.

QUESTIONS FOR REFLECTION

1. As a prospective client of a somatic practitioner (or other professional), has your decision regarding whether to make an appointment ever been strongly influenced, pro or con, by the practitioner's demeanor during the initial phone conversation? What made the difference?

2. Has the appearance of a manual therapist's office or work environment ever been off-putting for you? What made you uncomfortable?

3. In your work life, have you ever made an exception for a client or customer and then been sorry you did? What happened, and what motivated you to make that exception? What did you learn from that experience?

4. Why do you think we need consistency in this work?

5. Have you ever chosen one professional (or any kind of service person such as a plumber or car mechanic) over another because of their attention to framework details?

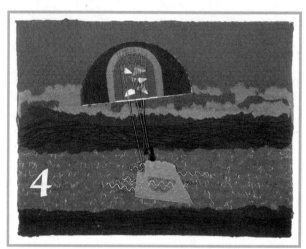

Chapter 4

CLIENT-PRACTITIONER DYNAMICS: BOUNDARIES AND THE POWER IMBALANCE

For a deeper understanding of the need for good boundaries and framework, we have to take a closer look at our relationships with clients. Often those relationships are more complicated than they appear at first. Much is going on beneath the surface that may seem puzzling and challenging, making it difficult for practitioners to stay clear headed and compassionate.

Clients respond to us in ways we can't always explain—sometimes they touch our hearts, and sometimes they push our buttons. Some clients act as if we're gods, and others seem monumentally unimpressed. Some are as open to us as children; others seem to be wearing a suit of armor. Sometimes we feel drained by clients, and other times, we feel exhilarated by them. Often we don't understand either reaction.

Transference and Countertransference

Understanding the built-in power difference between us and our clients is the key to unraveling the complexities of those relationships. We are more important to our clients than we often realize. When we take on the role of practitioner, it is that role, not necessarily who we are personally, that gives us special authority or power in clients' eyes.

For one thing, the intimacy of the situation may bring up unconscious issues for clients (and, as we will see later, for us as well). That holds true even if our work is not psychologically oriented, even if we are "just" giving a massage. On some level, those unconscious factors can tend to make clients feel dependent on us or even like children. Consider the circumstances that we work in: we are clothed, our clients are naked or close to it. We are active, they are relatively passive. What we are doing and why we are doing it are often unclear to them—not because we have not explained it well but because much of our work defies verbal explanation. Our touch is often nurturing, sometimes probing, but always personal. Also, clients (and practitioners) are often in an altered state of consciousness, a state in which they are less in their thinking minds and more open and vulnerable than they usually are in their day-to-day lives. Add these factors together, and we can begin to appreciate the strong influences going on during sessions.

It's natural for clients to experience us—again, on an unconscious level—as a parent or authority figure. In their minds, we become a little (or a lot) larger than life and more powerful than they are. Everyone has more or less unresolved issues related to parents or authority figures, and clients bring those issues into the session. Because of that, clients may look up to us with far more admiration than they would if they met us in another context. Or they may be more wary of us than they would ordinarily be.

Psychological theory calls the process of how clients react to the power imbalance **transference**. Old hurts, longings, and conflicts from a client's past relationships with authority figures or important others are unconsciously *transferred* to us in our role as practitioner. For instance, a client who was physically abused as a child may have an unconscious fear of being injured by the large person (and we all look big as we stand over clients) looming over him. Or the client who felt lonely and abandoned as a child may hope for his practitioner to be the all-giving, totally loving parent he wished he'd had.

Transference: When a client unconsciously projects (transfers) unresolved feelings, needs, and issues—usually from childhood and usually related to parent or other authority figures—onto a practitioner.

How do we know that transference is happening? Clients aren't usually consciously aware of these feelings, so they don't generally talk about them. Instead, we see transference in the ways clients relate to us. For instance, some clients defer to us and never question our judgment, others show adoration or develop crushes, and still others seem to mistrust us for no obvious reason. ("Crush" in this context describes a feeling of admiration for or attraction to a practitioner that is similar to the innocent feelings that a third grader has for his or her favorite teacher. Although there may be a hint of sexual feeling, the client doesn't attempt to act on it.)

What does transference mean to you in your role of being a caring practitioner? You will never understand all that is going on inside your clients, and you do not want to try to be their analyst. But you do need to know that the dynamics of your interactions with clients are more complex than they seem. You also need to know how to help clients feel safe with you in light of these dynamics.

Positive and Negative Transference

One way to look at transference is in terms of its positive and negative aspects.

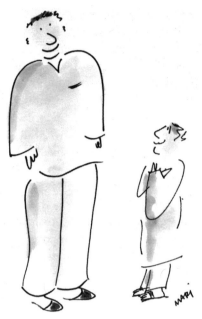

Positive transference.

POSITIVE TRANSFERENCE

We call it positive transference when a client has special affection or adoration or deference towards us. Clients can feel as if they are small and relatively insignificant and we are large and benevolent. We see this when clients have innocent crushes on us or are in awe of us and think we are special and wonderful.

NEGATIVE TRANSFERENCE

We see negative transference in clients who mistrust us without good reason, who expect us to hurt or criticize them. Here are two examples of negative transference:

> A new client is nervous and asks an unusual number of questions about the practitioner's qualifications. During the bodywork session, the client pulls back at the slightest hint of discomfort. Later, she reveals that she was physically abused as a child.

> A male client seems very "controlling," telling the practitioner exactly where and how deep he wants the work to be. He has a hard time relaxing, resists closing his eyes during a session, and is constantly aware of small sounds from the outside. After several sessions, the practitioner learns that the client grew up in a war-torn country and endured constant air raids and fear for his life.

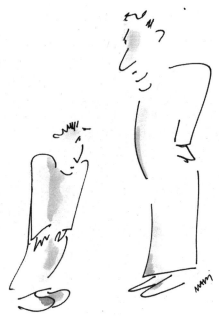

Negative transference.

Assuming that the practitioners in these examples provided safe, welcoming spaces and presented themselves as professional and attentive, these clients were not responding to the actual situation in front of them; the danger they were reacting to was in their past, not the present. It's not useful for practitioners to respond with annoyance or dismay when clients seem overly sensitive, try to take charge, or are especially vigilant. Understanding that unconscious fears may motivate such reactions helps us respond with compassion and attentiveness.

With negative transference—when the client is critical of us or doesn't trust us—we sometimes have the feeling of, "But I didn't do anything." Or "Why does that bother her? It doesn't bother anyone else." Although negativity from the client may feel like a threat or an attack, it is usually no more about us than are positive transference reactions. Human nature being what it is, we often see negative transference as the client's problem, as some kind of character defect, yet we see positive transference as a natural response to our winning personality or exceptional skills.

We can't always know what a client is feeling—or why. In fact, we may misinterpret a client's behavior; clients (and people in general) don't always act the way they feel. A client who feels afraid of us may act defiant. A client who thinks the practitioner is the best thing since sliced bread may act nonchalant. And to make it more complicated, clients often feel both positive and negative transference toward their practitioners. Whatever form the transference takes, be aware that clients are giving extra weight to what we say and do.

Transference, A Normal Process

Transference may sound complex and unusual, but it's actually part of our everyday life even outside our offices. It's normal for any of us to bring the past into our present relationships. In fact, it happens all the time:

> Mary overreacts to her boyfriend's teasing because her father, who teased her, was critical and hurtful in other ways.

> John feels especially connected to and possessive of a friend who is nurturing to him in a way that John's mother was not.

These kinds of transference are common in our everyday lives. But they are magnified in a manual therapy session because of the intimacy of the setting, the client's altered state, and the way that the practitioner/client roles mimic those of parent/child.

Once clients connect with us as practitioners, transference just happens. Never mind that our clients are adults or may even be older than we are. Transference isn't a rational process. It's more like the way baby ducks follow after the first animal they see. It has been many years since I had my first Rolfing series, but if my first Rolfer happened to walk by today, I would want to waddle after him, quacking and flapping.

Some well-meaning practitioners will protest, "But I want to be an equal with my clients. I don't want to have any power over them." Although this is a noble idea, transference can't be avoided. The situation isn't a level playing field from the outset. No matter what our good intentions, it's natural that some degree of transference happens.

The minute we take on a client, we acquire a responsibility toward that person. The relationship is unequal, and it is likely to continue that way for as long as we know the client. True, we want to continue to give power back to the client, as appropriate. Ways to do that are discussed later in this chapter.

Countertransference

Practitioners come to bodywork sessions with all their own history, too. Like clients, we are in an intimate situation and often in an altered state while

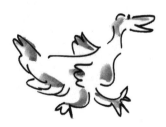

we work. In these conditions, practitioners also can lose their objectivity. Old feelings and attitudes can cloud our judgment and interfere with the way we respond to clients. When a practitioner transfers feelings to a client that belong in the practitioner's past or that are related to the practitioner's issues, it is called **countertransference**.

Countertransference, like transference, is an unconscious process—usually we're not consciously aware of why we're responding to a client in a certain way. Here are some possible scenarios that show countertransference:

> **Counter-transference:** When a practitioner allows unresolved feelings and personal issues to influence his relationship with a client.

> Massage therapist Martha responds with irritation to a picky, complaining client, who has made many requests. When the client makes one more request, this time for more heat, Martha snaps, "I hope this is the last request you'll make. I can't concentrate on my work."
>
> Although Martha's not aware of it, that client reminds her of her chronically complaining mother. Martha may think she's responding as any practitioner would to an annoying client. However, she's actually relating to the client as an angry child would. If Martha stepped back into her professional role, she might realize that the client has a right to ask for alterations that will help her comfort.

> Bodyworker Bill bends over backwards for his kindly older client, Robert, who acts as if everything Bill does is wonderful. In Bill's mind, Robert has become the ideal dad he longed for, so he makes extra concessions for Robert, scheduling sessions at times he doesn't usually work and extending credit when he usually requires payment with each session. When Robert doesn't respond as quickly to treatment as Bill wants him to, Bill feels crushed. He doesn't see that he's relating to the client as if he were a child wanting to do anything to please his parent. If Bill were being an objective professional, he wouldn't bend his boundaries without good reason, and he wouldn't be discouraged by the normal ups and downs of treatment.

> When a regular client decides to stop making appointments because his back doesn't hurt anymore, somatic practitioner Sue relates to the event as if the client were the parent who abandoned her. Sue feels angry and rejected rather than having the healthy perspective that she's done such good work that the client is now able to stop seeing her.

Transference and Countertransference Together

A client's emotional transference-driven response can elicit an emotional countertransference response from the practitioner. As an example, consider

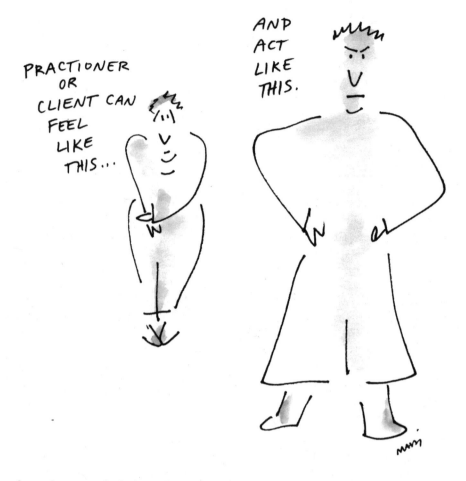

that when people feel small and defenseless, they may act angry and critical. A client who feels small and defenseless may react with anger or pickiness, and the practitioner, who then also feels small and defenseless, may react with irritation and defensiveness. Both the client and the practitioner feel threatened and end up acting critical or menacing.

Here's an example:

> Both client and practitioner are perfectionists—both believe that they never measured up to their parents' expectations, and both still carry that insecurity. The practitioner, meaning to give information and sympathy, says to the client, "Boy, you're tight in your upper back." The client hears it as a parental criticism of his ability to take care of himself and responds with an irritated, "That's what you're supposed to help me with!" The practitioner hears that as a criticism of her professional skills and mumbles an exasperated, "I'm doing the best I can."

A more therapeutic response from the practitioner might be to say cheerfully, "You're right—it *is* what I'm supposed to do! I meant to say that it looks like you've been under a good deal of stress."

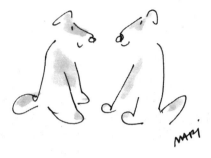

Signs of Transference

There are various ways that we can tell that positive or negative transference is in play.

Clients' Passivity

One sign that clients have promoted us to an elevated status is that they rarely express their unhappiness with something we're doing, and they often agree to something they don't really want to do. They may tell us, for instance, that they are fine lying in a position that is actually making their neck hurt. They often don't speak up when we make them uncomfortable, such as when we've set the room temperature too hot, we're talking too much, or even when they think we've crossed sexual boundaries. If we make them too uncomfortable, they simply don't come back, sometimes without being conscious of the reason. Or they might remain as clients but become what we call "difficult" clients.

The sense of powerlessness that usually goes with being a client is especially noticeable when the client is also a peer. I hear many stories from even seasoned practitioners who have had trouble speaking up when getting work on themselves. You would think that, as professionals, we would have no trouble asserting ourselves, but because of the power of the transference, because of what happens when *we* are on the table, we may be as speechless as anyone else. If we feel powerless to question our colleagues, how must our clients feel?

Here are stories told by practitioners who were the client at the time.

> The session ended 20 minutes earlier than usual, but I didn't question it.

> The gardener was cutting the grass with a loud lawn mower right outside the window, and it was hard to focus, but I didn't say anything.

> He expressed sexual interest in me during the session. He's such a nice guy that although I told him I wasn't interested, I didn't tell him how upset I was at his inappropriateness.

Practitioners who tell these stories are usually bewildered or embarrassed that they didn't speak up when they were the client. "I know I should have said something," they say apologetically.

Even in the most traumatizing situations—sexual violations—clients rarely assert themselves. There are many stories of a practitioner intentionally or unintentionally crossing a sexual boundary and then, when later confronted, protesting, "But she didn't say anything."

Sometimes power differences are exaggerated by circumstances that either give the practitioner extra authority or make the client more powerless. For instance, cultural perceptions about authority come into play. The authority gap can be greater when a man is working with a woman or when a practitioner is physically much larger than a client. Also, the power difference is exaggerated when a practitioner is a client's teacher or has special status in the community. It can also be heightened if we are working with a client in crisis.

> An experienced bodywork client who was having acute back spasms went to see a bodyworker who was esteemed in the community. The client said, "During the session, I felt like what she was doing wasn't right for me, but this woman is 'the best,' and I didn't question her. I ended up feeling injured by her work."

Practitioners who fit into any of these categories may need to take extra care to help their clients feel safe. For example, all of us need to explain what the treatment will involve, get clients' consent before treatment, and let clients know they have the right to refuse any part of the treatment or ask the practitioner to stop. However, for their own protection as well, practitioners who know the power imbalance is greater than usual will need to be especially alert to signs of discomfort in clients.

The Captive Audience

Positive transference can be so subtle and pervasive that we can take advantage of it without realizing it. For instance, during a session, we may talk on and on about our philosophy of life while the client listens as if to a great guru. Just because the client has fallen into the illusion that we are wiser and somehow better than they are doesn't mean that we have to fall right in there with them.

It can be appealing to have an attentive audience that defers to us. In the presence of the admiring (or, at least, not overtly complaining) client, we may imagine we have such interesting stories to tell or that our opinions and thoughts on just about anything are especially meaningful. When we allow that to happen, we have forgotten that the client is the star of the show, not us.

Clients may put up with practitioner's self-centeredness. Who would risk insulting someone who holds the key to helping or hindering them? Clients come to us hoping to feel better, and sometimes they are in pain. Who would risk offending their bodyworker?

When we mistake positive transference for the truth or when we buy into the illusion that we are somehow better than the client, we lose our curiosity about the client—and we lose our effectiveness. What are the client's strengths and dreams? What pain is the client ready to release? What does the client want from the session? Clients know more about themselves than we do—sometimes they simply don't know that they know. Our job is to help them find the best in themselves, not to impose our own needs and egos.

Our curiosity and compassion go out the window when we pretend to be all knowing or when we forget that the session belongs to the client. Even if clients need to put us on a pedestal, we have to find ways to let them know that, although we are competent, we are merely consultants who have certain gifts and training; they are the ones who have the power in their own lives.

Lost Souls

Isn't it okay to have some clients who really like us, clients with whom we have a great connection? The answer depends on another question: Are our sessions with them about us or about them? Are those clients lost souls coming to hear what we have to say, or are we the ones who listen with curiosity and interest to what they bring to a session?

Some clients try hard to please us, and that can feel good. But by basking in the glow of our own egos, we can miss the desperation underneath their efforts to please. Certified Feldenkrais trainer Paul Rubin talks about clients who are at a time in their lives when they feel like "lost souls:" "Many people are at a choice point of 'Do I find myself, or do I find someone I can see as more powerful with whom I can have a dependent relationship?' It's always up to us to guide people back to finding their independence."

It's natural and therapeutic for clients to be dependent and look up to us at certain times. Certainly, most of us have had times in our lives when we felt like lost souls. However, if our practices are full of people who call us after hours or who rely on us to help them make decisions, then we need to take a look at what's going on. Are we getting our own emotional needs met by cultivating dependency in clients? It's not our job to run our clients' lives. As a colleague, Janet Zimmerman, so aptly put it, "We have to remember that we're just the hired hands."

Sexual Feelings

Crushes are a common form of transference, and it is easy to think that they are about us. They really are not. (Again, we're not talking about clients who are sexually inappropriate or aggressive with us.) Crushes don't mean that clients want romantic relationships with their practitioners. Rather, the client's unconscious is using the practitioner (in an appropriate, therapeutic way) to deal with deep issues. For instance, they may see in us the good, nurturing parent they wish they'd had. Or maybe the work itself, the softening of tightly held tissue, has helped them get in touch with old longings, and they then think those longings have something to do with us. Our work with such clients, perhaps our acceptance of them, has awakened something in them, but their feelings aren't really about us.

Marion Rosen, founder of Rosen Method bodywork, uses the term "stand in" to describe what we are to our clients:

> I am 84 years old, and when a 30-year-old male client tells me he is in love with me, I tell him that this feeling has arisen in him from the work we are doing together and that I am just a "stand in" to enable him to do the inner work he needs to do.

If the client with a crush is of an age and gender we are usually attracted to, the situation can be more dangerous; it may make it easier both to misinterpret the client's intentions and to return the interest. Practitioners who are drawn to doing that should seek outside help to sort it out. It's unethical to take advantage of a client's romantic transference feelings for us.

How to Work With Transference

Many psychotherapists actively work with transference to help clients heal old wounds, learn new patterns of relating, and so forth. Although that is beyond our scope of practice, we can still be therapeutic in our actions. For instance, if a client is (unconsciously) expecting the worst, such as punishment or criticism, then it must surely be helpful for that client if the practitioner's responses are, instead, caring and reasonable. Or it can be helpful with a smitten client for the practitioner not to soak up the adulation, but instead, to gently give the power back to the client, as discussed later in this chapter. Some guidelines for dealing with transference are provided next.

DON'T TALK TO CLIENTS ABOUT THEIR TRANSFERENCE

The first rule is—and this is one of the rare times the word "rule" is used in this book—don't talk to clients about what you imagine their transference to be. For instance, don't say, "You're just upset with me because you're still mad at your mother" or "You have a crush on me because you need a strong father figure."

For one thing, you don't really know what's causing their behavior. For another, remember that transference is unconscious; the client may not know what you're talking about and may find it confusing or annoying. It can seem patronizing to tell clients your ideas about their motivations. It assumes both that you know more about them than they do and that you have license to talk about psychological dynamics with them. A client coming to us for a relaxing massage, a balancing structural integration session, or an enlivening hour of movement work probably doesn't have an interest in our psychological theories.

UNDERSTAND THAT TRANSFERENCE ISN'T USUALLY ABOUT YOU

It's worth saying this again: "Transference" means the client's reaction is only superficially about you. Whether it's adoration or deep mistrust, it's often not really about the practitioner. (Although there's probably a grain of truth behind their reaction—you've done something that pleases or displeases them—their response is out of proportion to the actual event.) Practitioners are mistaken if they think they really are that perfect when clients adore them or that awful when clients are mad at them.

Clients may want to take care of you, please you, challenge you, or berate you. None of these responses is necessarily about you. The challenge is to keep an even keel and not be swayed by clients' reactions.

Practitioners are mistaken if they think they really are that perfect when clients adore them or that awful when clients are mad at them.

KNOW WHEN TRANSFERENCE IS ABOUT YOU

Knowing the dynamics of transference, however, doesn't give you license to dismiss all clients' complaints or criticisms as simply their old unresolved issues. If you keep getting the same kinds of negative feedback, it probably *is* about you. Understanding transference should make practitioners more respectful of and sensitive to clients.

There's truth in both positive and negative transference, but that truth is usually about your professional self, not your private self. Clients who love you may be responding to the fact that, during your sessions with them, you are caring, concerned, and sensitive to their needs. However, if clients knew you in your personal life, they would have a fuller, more human, and less idealized picture. By the same token, a client who has trouble trusting you may be responding to a problem with your professional behavior, not who you are in your private life. For instance, if you were chronically late in starting sessions, clients for whom punctuality is important might see you as an uncaring and inconsiderate person, regardless of whether that is generally true about you.

KEEP THE BOUNDARIES EXTRA CLEAR

Faced with a strong negative or positive transference, your job is to be extra crisp about boundaries and to pay close attention to framework. If the client is already in "transference" love with you, for example, you would not want to accept her invitation to a party or in any way encourage a more social relationship. If the client is already uncomfortable with you, taking even greater care with the therapeutic environment can help her feel safer. The more you keep boundaries clear, the less chance that transference will become destructive to the therapeutic relationship.

BE RESPECTFUL

Whether they exhibit crushes or fears, all clients deserve practitioners' respect, not their judgments. We don't know where any of these feelings originate in clients. We don't know what their histories are or what deep aspects have been stirred. A colleague tells this story:

A client complained about being poked by my fingernails, and I debated a minute before deciding to do anything about them. I'd just gotten a manicure—lovely red nails—and I'd just seen my favorite teacher, who also had long nails, work without pain to her client. Nevertheless, I decided to file my nails and was glad I did. Later in the session, my client told me that when she was a child, her mother would punish her by actually cutting her skin with her long red fingernails.

DON'T TAKE ADVANTAGE OF CLIENTS

Avoid taking advantage of clients' transference even in small ways, such as using them as an easy audience. Practitioners who use the affection that clients have for them for their own advantage—trying to turn a client into a business or romantic partner, for example—are committing the worst kind of ethical violation.

KEEP GIVING THE POWER BACK

By your behavior, you can let clients know that this is a therapeutic situation—that you aren't an abusive parent *or* a savior and that the power is in their hands. Sometimes you can tell them these things directly with phrases such as, "You're the expert on your own body" or "Please tell me if you want me to stop what I'm doing at any time."

From your first interview, let them know that you are working with them in partnership. Ask them what they want from their work with you and explain your work as carefully as possible so that they know what is being offered to them. Let them know that you won't take it personally if they want changes in the environment or the work itself—for instance, if they want you to turn the heat up or down or work more lightly or more deeply. Avoid treating them like children or creating your own agenda for them. Here's an example:

A client came to a practitioner for a relaxing massage for her sore back. Without asking the client her wishes, the practitioner decided that the client also needed to do exercises at home and sent her home with instructions. The practitioner was then upset when the client returned and had not done her "homework."

Think in terms of educating and suggesting rather than imposing and ordering.

Signs of Countertransference

Countertransference happens when practitioners bring unresolved issues and feelings into the session. When you take what a client says or does personally, it is considered countertransference. For instance, if you're constantly disappointed and angry with uncooperative clients, that's a red flag. What you can reasonably expect from clients is some form of payment and that they treat you with respect. As long as they aren't abusively insulting or disrespectful, clients should be free to complain, become enamored of you, improve, not improve, and generally go at their own pace without your taking it personally. If you expect certain kinds of validation—that they get better at a certain rate so you can feel like a "good" practitioner or that they praise your work during every session—that is countertransference and is not useful.

The intimacy of bodywork triggers deep emotions and old feelings, and practitioners are as much a part of that unconscious soup as are clients. Practitioners can easily lose their objectivity. Any strong feelings about a client—anger, chronic annoyance, or even love or caring—can signal that you are lost in countertransference. Another common red flag for countertransference is feeling tired or drained when you work with certain clients. Be curious about any negative reactions to clients and get help with understanding these feelings.

What about being fond of your clients? Isn't it natural that you open your heart to your clients? One way to distinguish healthy from unhealthy affection for clients is the extent to which they have become "special" to you. Do you give extra attention to what you're wearing if you're seeing them that day? Do you make exceptions for them that you don't for other clients? Do you give them extra time, rearrange your schedule to accommodate them, or let their bills slide? Do you go out of your way to help them with an outside problem? In other words, do you bend your own boundaries for this client?

A colleague relates:

> I was attracted to one of my new clients and at first wasn't conscious of it. After a few sessions, I began to have signs of countertransference: I always looked forward to her session with some excitement and felt "high" at the end. I made a point of telling her about upcoming events that might be of interest to her and realized that this was in hopes that I might "accidentally" bump into her. She had a busy work life, and I often came in earlier than I usually do to accommodate her. After I became aware of what I was doing, I discussed the attraction with a professional consultant and was able to regain my balance with this client.

If you imagine that you are the only one who can truly understand or help a particular client, you are headed for trouble. If you see yourself as "rescuing" a poor, helpless client, that's a red flag, too.

As for negative countertransference, aren't some people just annoying? Perhaps. But it also could be that another practitioner would find them endearing, or it could be that your "annoying client" is simply anxious or even responding to your careless framework. Do you think a particular client got

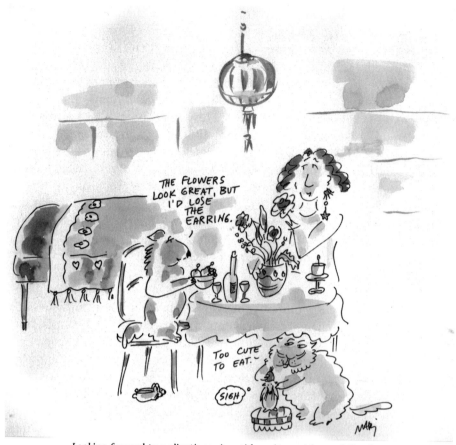

Looking forward to a client's session with excitement is a red flag for countertransference issues.

up that morning with the intention of irritating you and making your day seem longer? Or do you sense that that is generally the way she copes with situations that are difficult for her?

Clients who seem difficult or demanding are often trying to mask their underlying fear, neediness or confusion. The helpful response to these clients is actually just the opposite of our natural inclination. Most of us would be naturally inclined to be impatient and have a "get-over-it" attitude with such a client. However, to really settle this client down, we can respond with attentiveness and concern, for instance, to ask for extra feedback about whether she is comfortable—how's the room temperature, does she want a deeper or lighter pressure, what else does she need to help her relax? It's easy to be caring with an appreciative client; picky clients are the true test of our compassion.

It's easy to be caring with an appreciative client; picky clients are the true test of our compassion.

How to Work With Countertransference

Countertransference happens constantly. It's not a question of "if," but rather of when and how it arises and what kind of people you most easily overreact to. And after you think you've got your inner responses to clients figured out, someone walks through the door who turns you upside down, who makes you wonder why you feel mad, fascinated, or exhausted. Working with your own transference (which is called countertransference) is an ongoing learning process.

NOTICE WHEN YOU MAKE EXCEPTIONS

As discussed earlier, one of the best ways to know when you are acting out of countertransference is to notice when you want to go outside your usual boundaries or change the usual structure of your sessions. When you come in an hour earlier than usual for a client, are you responding to a real need? Or are you accommodating him because you feel too intimidated, guilty, or perhaps charmed to ask the client to fit into your schedule? Paying attention to framework and boundaries provides safety for you because countertransference just naturally happens. We're all human and always have unresolved issues, old wounds, and insecurities that color our judgments.

GET OUTSIDE HELP

After you have identified your own countertransference, then you can figure out how best to work with it. Sometimes just being aware of it is enough to overcome it. However, other times, you need to get outside help with both recognizing it and learning how to turn those feelings into a better understanding of the client and of yourself. A good way to learn how to recognize when a client hooks you is to consult with a professional trained in psychological dynamics—a counselor or psychotherapist, for instance. Such consultation can help illuminate your countertransference and deal with your feelings related to your clients' transference.

> A practitioner found herself unusually annoyed with a client—a woman who was slightly older than the practitioner and who seemed sweet but passive. In talking with her supervisor, the practitioner realized that the client reminded her of her mother's passivity, which often angered her. Once she realized that her feelings were related more to her mother than to her client, she was able to work with that client more objectively.

Talking over your responses to clients with a consultant can help you gain the objectivity you need to be skilled in your client relationships. Some practitioners prefer having an ongoing supervisory relationship with a consultant for support and help with identifying their strengths and weaknesses in relationships with clients. A supervisor can help you know, for instance, when it may be appropriate to refer a client to someone else. If you've done your best to find compassion for a client but are still constantly irritated, you're not helping such a client by continuing to work with him or her. Likewise, if you've discussed your feelings of attraction to a client and those feelings are still intruding into a session, you need to refer that client to another practitioner. It is against professional ethics to work with clients toward whom you have strong feelings of either attraction or repulsion.

Practitioners who regularly consult with professional counselors or bodyworkers trained in psychological dynamics find that it helps them sort out these issues and makes their jobs easier. Strong positive or negative feelings about a client are red flags. Getting outside help can turn those annoyances or infatuations into solid learning experiences.

Hearts and Minds

Giving and receiving bodywork can both touch our hearts and cloud our minds. Bodywork brings up unconscious material—for our clients as well as ourselves—that can interfere with the therapeutic relationship. Clients get mad at us, clients fall in love with us, and we get irritated or love them back. Our role is to sort out those feelings in a way that empowers our clients and helps them heal old wounds. Our job is to do our best to keep our own issues from intruding into the therapeutic process.

Clear boundaries and a sturdy framework help both parties handle their transference and countertransference reactions. They orient us and bring clarity to the murkiness that arises from unresolved personal history. When we strive to be consistent and even handed, we can identify our red flags more quickly and get help when heading down the wrong path. It takes careful thought, training, and determination not to let the power imbalance inherent in the therapeutic relationship throw us off.

Appreciating the power of transference and countertransference is the key to understanding why we need to take care with boundaries and framework. In fact, the power imbalance between client and practitioner is the reason for most professional rules of ethics. Without an understanding of those dynamics, ethical and boundary guidelines can seem like arbitrary dictates rather than necessary structure.

QUESTIONS FOR REFLECTION

1. Think of a situation when you were the client of a manual therapist (or other practitioner) when the practitioner was doing something that you didn't agree with or that was making you uncomfortable. Did you question the practitioner at the time or assert yourself? If you did assert yourself, did something that the practitioner said or did make it easy for you to do so? If you didn't, what could he or she have done to make it easier?

2. As an adult, have you ever greatly admired someone who was in a professional role with you? How did the professional handle it? What was helpful or not helpful in the way the professional responded to your admiration?

3. Have you ever felt small or helpless with an authority figure or a practitioner and then acted "big" and angry? What other ways do you react in the presence of an authority figure?

4. Can you think of a recent time in your everyday life when your response to someone may have come from old perceptions or patterns (transference) rather than the reality of the moment?

5. Have you ever had a manual therapist or practitioner use you as a captive audience? How did you feel? If you didn't like it, did you express that at the time?

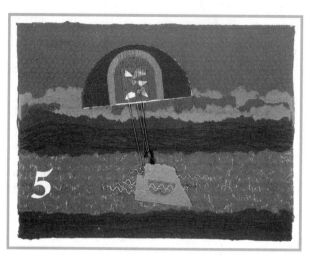

Chapter 5

*E*THICAL BOUNDARIES: FROM THEORY TO PRACTICE

We can look for simple answers about ethics—what are the rules, and how do we stay out of trouble? However, there are few black-and-white absolutes to which we can cling. To make wise decisions, we usually have to thread our way through the gray and uncertain areas of the therapeutic relationship with all its details and nuances, its transference and countertransference issues. Also, to decide the right thing to do, we have to consider not only the details of the particular situation but also the broader picture of how an action will affect our clients, our own reputation, and the reputation of our profession.

Ethical Questions

The following questions will help you determine whether an action may lead you down the wrong path. They can help you avoid harm to clients, to your relationship with clients, and to your reputation and the reputation of the profession.

- Would this action take advantage of the power, affection, or goodwill that clients give me because of my role (transference)?
- Would it violate the client's privacy or confidentiality?
- Would this action create a dual relationship (a relationship with the client outside that of client and practitioner) and, therefore, make the professional relationship less clear?

- Would it exceed the boundaries of the original implied contract—going beyond either my area of expertise or what the client has agreed upon?
- Would it be an exception to my usual policies?
- Regardless of how an action appears to me or my client, would it look inappropriate to others?
- Would the action be disrespectful of the client?

It may be obvious why some of these questions are included and less apparent why others are. Let's take a closer look at these questions, grouped by their ethical intentions.

Protecting Clients' Vulnerability

- Would this action take advantage of the power, affection, or goodwill that clients give you because of your role (transference)?
- Does it violate the client's privacy or confidentiality?

Most ethical standards are aimed at keeping practitioners from taking advantage of the power difference between them and their clients—using a client's affection and goodwill to benefit themselves personally.

Respecting clients' privacy and confidentiality is also a central part of what it means to be professional and to be sensitive to a client's vulnerability.

You can overstep boundaries in small ways that seem harmless—for instance, taking advantage of transference by talking too much during a session or breaching confidentiality by advising someone who has referred a client that the client has made an appointment. However, the more disciplined you are in honoring the boundaries of transference and confidentiality in even small ways, the less likely you are to err in more serious ways.

Most ethical standards are aimed at keeping practitioners from taking advantage of the power difference between them and their clients—using a client's affection and goodwill to benefit themselves personally.

Keeping Small Boundary Mistakes From Leading to Big Problems

- Would this action create a dual relationship and, therefore, make the professional relationship less clear?
- Would it exceed the boundaries of the original implied contract—going beyond either your area of expertise or what the client has agreed upon?
- Would it be an exception to your usual policies?

Significant ethical mistakes rarely come out of the blue. These questions relate to the fact that the more you bend boundaries, the more likely you are to get into serious ethical problems. Many boundary transgressions, such as having dual relationships with clients, aren't necessarily unethical by themselves, but they can become bigger problems if you make a habit of doing them without being alert to the difficulties.

A massage therapist who often socialized with her clients had a hard time keeping her roles straight. One of the clients she socialized with had told the massage therapist during a session that she had multiple sclerosis (MS) and wanted to keep it a secret. However, one day, another friend was criticizing that client and the massage therapist said, "Don't be so hard on her. She has MS." The client with MS found out about the confidentiality violation and, understandably outraged, filed an ethics complaint against the therapist with her professional association. A breach of confidentiality that would have been disturbing enough had it simply occurred between friends became a violation for which there were serious professional consequences for the massage therapist.

Avoiding the Appearance of Inappropriateness or Impropriety

- Regardless of how an action appears to you or your client, would it look inappropriate to others?

"Impropriety" may sound like a prim and proper word to the often free-spirited members of this profession. As long as you know you're a good, conscientious professional, you may not want to concern yourself with how something looks to an outsider or, in effect, what the neighbors think. However, you can't ignore the fact that massage continues to be linked in the public's mind to sexual services. Although it's unfortunate that our culture often equates nudity and touch with sexual behavior, that's the reality that you have to live with. It's not fair that the manual therapy profession is sometimes misjudged or that good professionals sometimes have to contend with offensive assumptions, but if you want to help your own reputation and that of the profession, it's best to be cautious.

Consider these statements from well-meaning massage therapists:

I tell my clients that as long as they're comfortable with it, they don't have to be draped.

I'm interested in dating Bob, so I invited him to come to my office and get a free massage. Since it's free, it doesn't affect my professional image.

You can imagine how these situations could have a negative effect on the reputation of both the professional and the profession. Suppose a prospective client heard that a massage therapist doesn't require draping. It could color this person's opinion of the massage therapist and, if he wasn't familiar with the fact that draping is supposed to be a standard protocol of massage, could color his opinion about all massage therapists.

In the second example, bringing a social and possible sexual element into your work and into your office—off-hours or not—is a bad idea. It can give the client or anyone who hears about it the idea that you regularly mix your romantic life with your work.

You should not give people any room for their imaginations to run away with them. Maybe an action seems innocent to you and to the client involved, but how will it look to the public? Your colleagues won't appreciate it if you lower the reputation of massage therapy and bodywork in the community. It means they will have the indignity of fielding more phone calls from prospective clients who expect sexual services; they will have the annoyance and perhaps danger of more clients who arrive in their offices anticipating sexual relief; and they will have to endure more rolled eyes when they tell others what they do for a living. Why risk offending colleagues and promoting harmful misconceptions about the profession?

None of us works in a vacuum. Whether practitioners belong to a professional association or not, their behavior reflects on the profession and the other practitioners in their community. It's safest to be above reproach. Behave in such a manner that your friends and colleagues would feel comfortable sending you both their elderly aunt and their teenage son or daughter.

Behave in such a manner that your friends and colleagues would feel comfortable sending you both their elderly aunt and their teenage son or daughter.

Respecting Clients' Dignity

- Would the action be disrespectful of the client?

Consider these cases:

> The client of a deep tissue bodyworker left a message on the bodyworker's answering machine after his first session, complaining that the pain in his back had gotten worse since the session. The bodyworker decided that the client must be a chronic complainer and a nuisance and never returned his call.

> A massage therapist's client complained that she still had discomfort in her knees even though she had been coming for regular massages for weeks. The practitioner curtly responded, "If you'd lose some weight and get off the sofa and exercise, you might feel a lot better."

Generally, it's easy to treat clients with respect if they are appreciative and pleasant. Clients such as the two above, who complain or are demanding, are the ones who are most likely to try your patience and test your professional diplomacy. As a professional, you are obligated to respond to complaints with kindness or at least with civility. Even if a client is being abusive, it's unethical for practitioners to be rude or insulting.

Clients don't have a right to be personally insulting, call you names, or use harsh or vulgar language. (Of course, they also don't have a right to be physically threatening or sexually inappropriate.) However, they do have a right to complain about your work or question your professional knowledge, and you want to be able to respond to their concerns with care and objectivity. Complainers usually need education and reassurance. Depending on the situation, the client whose back was still hurting might need to hear, for instance, that it often takes a day or two before a client feels relief from pain. Or with the client whose knees still hurt, you could let her know you're on her side: "I'm sorry you're still having discomfort. Massage therapy often relieves joint pain, and I was hoping that it would help you."

Maintaining a good professional relationship with your clients also goes a long way toward keeping you out of major trouble. A small complaint handled poorly can balloon into a big problem; angry clients sometimes air their grievances in the community or, at the extreme, take them to your professional association or even to court.

Judgment Calls

We want to follow the standards of our state and national associations, but sometimes those standards are so generalized that it's difficult to know what they mean in practice. The goal is to learn how to make smart and ethical choices under any circumstance.

In any practice, certain situations require judgment calls on the part of practitioners who want to protect their clients, the profession, and their own reputations. Keeping in mind the questions and considerations already discussed, here are some examples of how to make good choices and judgment calls.

Sexual Relationships

THE ETHICAL STANDARD

It is unethical to have a sexual relationship with a client. With an ex-client, it is unethical to use the affection, power, or intimacy of the client-practitioner relationship to create a sexual relationship. It is also unethical to sexualize the relationship with a client by dressing seductively, flirting, or making remarks that could be construed as sexual.

JUDGMENT CALLS

> At a party, you are talking with someone you have just met, someone you find attractive. The person learns that you are a bodyworker (or massage therapist or movement teacher) and wants to make an appointment. Do you make the appointment?

> You have been working with a client for several months, and you re-
> alize that you are starting to feel sexually attracted to him or her.
> What do you do?

Everyone should know that the absolute rule is not to date or have sexual relations with a client, but what about sexual attractions? The answer
depends, for one thing, on how attracted you are:

- Is it just a passing thought?
- Is there a spark of sexual connection between you?
- Are you often aware of being sexually attracted to another person, or
  is this a rare feeling, so that the attraction takes on greater meaning?
- Are you feeling emotionally off kilter, so that you might be more than
  usually tempted to act on an attraction?
- Are you feeling open to a new attraction, even though you are mar-
  ried or in a relationship?
- Has it been your experience that you can be mildly attracted to a
  client without its interfering with your work?

You have to know yourself and your limitations. Sessions should always
focus on the client and not on your personal needs. If you have strong romantic or sexual feelings about a client, the feelings usually intrude into the
professional relationship. A strong attraction is a good issue to take to a
consultant or supervisor for discussion.

You should also consider the effect of transference. The decision to become someone's practitioner shouldn't be made casually. When someone
becomes a client (and often before he or she arrives on the table), transference begins and feelings are heightened on both sides. In the client's eyes,
you have already started to become a little larger than life—the compassionate caregiver, the heroic reliever of pain, or the nurturing parent figure.
Under these circumstances, clients are not as free to refuse romantic invitations. It's unethical to take advantage of this vulnerability.

Once someone becomes a client, you may never be able to have a normal social relationship with that person. The effects of transference are simply too deep. Once you become a person's practitioner, you have limited the
relationship. Most associations' ethics standards require that practitioners
wait at least 6 months before dating an ex-client. Regardless of the number
of months that have passed, practitioners dating an ex-client would be a
cause for concern and perhaps scrutiny in their professional circles. You're
better off deciding from the beginning whether a relationship will be professional or social.

Let's look back at the two examples. In the first example, how do you decide whether to make the appointment? To start with, it's never a good idea to
make an appointment or do business at a party. Just offer the person your
business card. That would also give you time to sort out your feelings, either

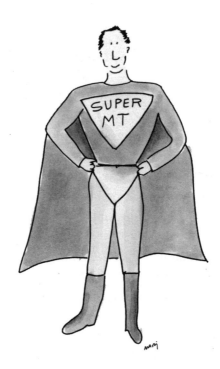

on your own or with outside help. If you know you're not in danger of acting on your sexual attraction, you can take the person as a client, knowing that you are thereby eliminating the possibility of having a sexual relationship with him while he is a client and possibly forever. If you're not sure whether you want to exclude that possibility, it's smart to buy time. For instance, when the person calls, you can simply say you don't have any appointments available and tell him to call back after a certain time. Given enough time, you can find your ethical bearings and decide whether to take that person as a client.

In the second situation, in which the practitioner becomes attracted to someone who is already a client, it's probably best to seek out help before making a decision about whether to continue to work with that client. As previously noted, any time you have strong feelings about a client, whether it's strong attraction or strong dislike, it's a good idea to talk with someone trained in psychological dynamics to help you sort it out. If you come to understand the reasons for the attraction, the feelings may dissipate. If they don't, then you probably need to stop working with the client. There's no set way to deal with either situation; each calls for a careful examination of the strength and motivation of your feelings and of what is best for that particular client. Such a judgment call can best be made with outside help.

Negative Judgments

THE ETHICAL STANDARD

We owe clients our care and attention. We may not connect with a person right away, but if we can't imagine ever having a caring attitude toward a particular client, we shouldn't work with him or her. We need to be on the alert for anything that interferes with our ability to touch a client in a respectful, nonjudgmental way. We are not just touching bodies—we're touching spirits.

JUDGMENT CALLS

> Your new client reveals that he belongs to a group that offends your belief system (for instance, he is a member of the National Rifle Association, a gay rights advocate, a fundamentalist, or pro-choice). Or he belongs to a group about whom you have general prejudgments (prejudices).

> Your client does something you find very annoying. For example, she talks constantly, never talks, has a whiny voice, or talks very loudly. You find yourself dreading her sessions.

Everyone prejudges other people. It's common for people to make snap judgments based on how people look, the way they dress, or their beliefs. No one is completely untouched by negative attitudes about groups of people that they may have been taught as children—whether by the family, the community, or society at large. In addition, everyone has personal likes and dislikes. The question is how much these negative feelings interfere with your work.

Working with people you don't care for can seriously compromise the safety of the therapeutic environment. You may be inclined to be late, to be less than present, to tune them out, to shortchange them on time, or to lack compassion. Practitioners cannot totally hide their personal feelings from clients. What client wants to be touched by uncaring hands?

Regarding the first example of a client who belongs to a group that you have judgments about, you want to decide what is best for the client. You must first be honest with yourself about your own prejudices. If you have a thought such as, "Uh oh, here's one of those kinds of people. They are all so lazy/immoral/rigid," do you believe the statement to be true? Or do you recognize it for what it is—a stereotype that may or may not be true for the individual in front of you? As professionals, we are obligated to come to our sessions with an open mind, and usually opening our minds takes some effort.

As professionals, we are obligated to come to our sessions with an open mind, and usually opening our minds takes some effort.

The same holds true for a client you may find annoying or dislike for no good reason—that is, the client isn't being abusive or disrespectful. You have to try to find something in you that connects with that person, something you can open your heart to.

If soul-searching doesn't work and your negative feelings are so intense that you can't find compassion for a client, then you need to suggest that the client see someone else. However, even if you refer that client on, once you have identified your own feelings of prejudice or personal dislike, then you are obligated to find a way to work through those feelings, perhaps with the help of a mentor or consultant.

How to discontinue working with a client is discussed later in this chapter. However, even before your relationship with a client gets under way, you can make it clear that either party can bow out at any time. Nan Narboe, a psychotherapist who supervises massage therapists and bodyworkers, suggests one way to make it easier:

> When you make the first appointment, tell your prospective client that the first few sessions will allow the client to decide whether she or he can effectively work with you and also allow you to decide whether your work is the most effective for this client. If you decide that you should not continue working with the client, you can then say, "I don't think my work will be as beneficial for you as X or Y" (other methods or other practitioners).

Taking Financial Advantage of a Client

THE ETHICAL STANDARD

It is unethical to use the privilege of the client-practitioner relationship to profit financially beyond our fee-for-service charges. It is not ethical to exploit the relationship by using it to influence the client to buy a product or service or to make any investment.

JUDGMENT CALLS

> Your friend is a distributor for a supplement you believe is of high quality and that is said to boost energy and help certain physical problems. You have taken these vitamins and feel very enthusiastic about their value. Your friend encourages you to become a distributor and sell them to your clients.

Is it ethical to sell products to a client? Some professional bodywork associations ban their members from doing so. Others don't put restrictions on this practice. Some practitioners have no qualms about selling vitamins, lotions, or magnets to clients. Others don't think it's a good idea. How do you decide what is right?

Looking back at the list of questions that you want to keep in mind, you can probably see a number of potential problems with selling goods to clients. The main ethical issue isn't whether it may benefit the client to use the product that you sell, it's whether you are unfairly using the power of the therapeutic relationship. Is the client really free to refuse, or would she make a purchase mainly to please you? Even if a massage therapist merely has products on display, a client could get the idea that it would please the practitioner if she bought them. Aside from the ethical considerations, even subtly attempting to sell products to clients could make some clients feel pressured and uncomfortable.

Another issue is that selling anything to a client other than the professional services you have contracted for creates a dual relationship, which is inherently problematic because it complicates the interaction between you and the client. Suppose a client to whom you have sold vitamins doesn't benefit as much as you led her to expect. That could damage your working relationship.

If clients are interested in a particular product, you can refer them to someone else. In this situation, there is no harm as long as you don't benefit financially from the referral or talk clients into trying the product.

Refusing to Work With a Client or Stopping Work With a Client

THE ETHICAL STANDARD

Practitioners have a right of refusal. We have a right to refuse to work with a prospective client or to discontinue working with a client if we think that we cannot form a therapeutic alliance with that client or if we do not have the training or physical capabilities to work with that client.

JUDGMENT CALLS

> Your regular client arrives, having spent the afternoon doing yard work, and is uncharacteristically dirty and sweaty.

> You have worked with a couple on outcall basis several times. While you are alone with the husband, he makes suggestive remarks.

> You weigh 100 pounds. Your prospective client weighs twice that and has requested deep work.

There are many reasons you may choose not to work with a client. Poor hygiene, inappropriate sexual behavior, or a physical mismatch for you are three reasons. There are other reasons a client may not be appropriate for your work or may be beyond your abilities. They may be mentally ill or may have physical conditions that make the kind of work you do unsuitable for them. You want to be aware of what those conditions are and of what your own physical and emotional limitations are.

In addition to not taking on clients with conditions that aren't appropriate for your kind of work, you also may want to limit the number of

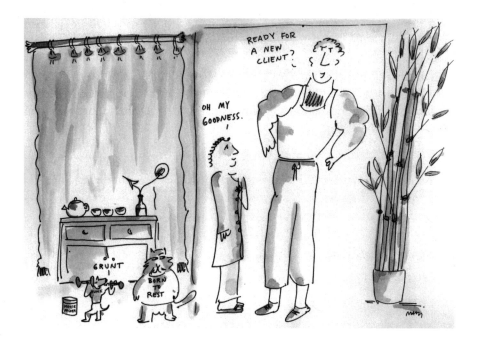

clients you see who present special difficulties, whether emotional or physical. These include clients who need extra help or reassurance and who take extra time in terms of phone calls and consultations outside their sessions; clients who are in acute physical distress; and clients who are beyond your physical capabilities, who are too large or densely muscled for you to work with effectively. You need to be aware of the limits of your skill and your physical abilities; it is unethical to take on clients you know you cannot serve well.

Regarding the situation with the sweaty client, most practitioners probably wouldn't mind working with an occasionally grimy client. Those who do mind need to make their policies clear up front to avoid the embarrassment of turning away a client. Spelling out these policies on an intake application form is a good way to get the point across. For instance, some massage therapy clinics post a notice or have clients sign a statement that says the therapists can refuse to work with someone or can terminate work because of a client's poor hygiene or inappropriate sexual behavior or comments.

In the case of the husband who made inappropriate remarks, it depends on your prior relationship with that person and the degree of offensiveness of the remarks. If, for instance, a client makes obvious offensive or degrading remarks, you should stop working with him at once—both stop the session and decline to make another appointment. If you are not clear about the person's intent or think he may just be testing you, you can give him a warning that you will not continue working with him unless he stops being suggestive. (Exceptions can be made for a regular client who makes a sexually oriented joke that's clearly not meant to be disrespectful and that doesn't offend you.) In this case, if the husband had never been inappropriate before, you could say, "I don't work with clients who don't treat me with respect. I'll end the massage if you make any more remarks like that." If he continues, you need to end the massage and let him know you won't work with him again. You might lose the wife's business also, but there's never a good reason to work with a disrespectful client.

When you decide not to take on someone who taxes your physical capabilities, you can be straightforward about your reasons: "I can't do justice to someone your size. May I give you the names of some practitioners who would be more appropriate?"

Sometimes you may not want to work with clients because they have emotional needs that you are not trained to handle—perhaps they are deeply depressed or working with issues of childhood abuse. Even if clients are working with a psychotherapist, you may still feel you would not be suited to work with them; for instance, you may feel overwhelmed about working with someone who cries a good deal. If these clients are not working with a psychotherapist, you have two choices: you can agree to work with the clients (not with their emotional issues but just as a massage therapist) with the understanding that they will seek psychological counseling as well, or you could let them know that you would be glad to refer them to a counselor or psychotherapist. Either way, you want to let these clients know that you do not have psychological training and that an experienced psychotherapist is usually the best help for the kinds of difficulties they are experiencing.

Confidentiality

THE ETHICAL STANDARD

Nothing a client says or does—and no information we have about a client—should be revealed to others without the client's permission unless disclosure is required by law or court order or is necessary for the protection of the public. Situations in which we can—and, in fact, are often obligated to—legally breach confidentiality are those in which there is clear and imminent danger to the client or others, there is suspicion of abuse or neglect of a child or incapacitated person, or there is a medical emergency.

JUDGMENT CALLS

Specific procedures for keeping patient information private are discussed in Chapter 3. However, practitioners can too easily violate confidentiality if they aren't careful.

For instance, in the situation with the husband who made sexually inappropriate remarks, what do you say to his wife if you decide not to continue to work with the husband? She's your client also, and you've been scheduling their appointments back to back at their home. The standards of confidentiality dictate that if the wife asks why you stopped seeing her husband, you can't tell her the reason. You can't even imply or suggest it. You have to say, "Even though he is your husband, I can't ethically talk about another client." If you've told her about your standards at the outset, it makes reinforcing the policy easier.

Violations of confidentiality can happen quickly. Here's an example: Mary and Susie are friends, and both are clients of Joe, a massage therapist. Mary says to Joe, "I haven't seen Susie in a while. How's she doing?" It's easy for Joe to say, "Oh, she's still having a hard time with her marriage." But if he does, he's broken confidentiality with Susie. To make it worse, now Mary knows that Joe passes on clients' private information to other people. Even "Susie's feeling great" is a violation. To keep clear framework, Joe can say lightly, "Oh, you know I can't talk about my other clients." Clients who are friends with other clients may sometimes test you—usually not consciously—to see if you will talk about their friend to them (and, therefore, talk to the friend about them).

Here's another way that practitioners can easily violate confidentiality. Quite often, if one client has referred a friend who then also becomes a client, the practitioner thanks the referrer, thereby letting him know that his friend is now a client. Although this is a common practice and it seems both harmless and good business manners to express gratitude, you might want to rethink it. Doesn't it violate the new client's privacy? Or a client says, "I told Dave about you. Did he ever call?" You want to thank the client for making the referral, but you shouldn't reveal whether Dave called or not. Just because the client made a referral, Dave's interactions with you don't become his business. You can say, "I appreciate your referral, and I understand why you want to know if he followed up. However, all my interactions with clients are confidential, so I can't tell you whether Dave called or not." When you first talk with a prospective client who has been referred by a friend or another client, you can ask permission to thank the friend for the referral.

Clients may want to keep the fact that they are seeing a manual therapist private for all kinds of reasons, such as not wanting to let their spouse know how they are spending money or fearing that someone else might think having a massage is a shady or self-indulgent practice.

If you see clients (past or present) in an outside setting, standard protocol is to not be the first to approach. Some clients may not have told their friends or family that they are seeing a massage therapist, and they may not want to have to explain who you are to their companion. If they acknowledge you, then you can match their level of friendliness. For instance, if a client merely nods to you, you can nod back but don't engage her in conversation. Even if the client is alone, she may not want to have her privacy invaded.

There are no exceptions to confidentiality. Sometimes you may be tempted to name-drop when a well-known or famous person is or has been a client. Famous people appreciate their privacy and have a right to it. Name-dropping is rarely impressive and only reveals the practitioner as someone who does not safeguard clients' privacy.

There's another aspect of confidentiality that relates to your own self-care. Amrita Daigle, a Trager Approach instructor, has noted that it can be difficult to maintain confidentiality unless we have a legitimate outlet for the feelings that build up in us during the work week. Many of us need a way to deal with the emotional stories that people tell us. Daigle suggests that we find a healthy outlet for our feelings, such as drawing, dancing, or meditating, and use it regularly. Consultants or supervisors, as described earlier, are also excellent and appropriate outlets. Getting ongoing body-work for yourself also helps with emotional overload.

However, talking with friends or colleagues about clients as a way of venting, even if you don't use names, isn't a good idea. The possibility of giving away information or identifying a client by accident is too great.

Other Ethical Standards and Implementation

Some ethics guidelines are fairly straightforward; we just need help with implementing them.

False Claims

THE ETHICAL STANDARD

Making false claims or inflated promises is unethical. It is unethical to obtain clients by persuasion or influence or to use comments about our services that contain untrue statements. It is unethical to create inflated or unjustified expectations of favorable results.

IMPLEMENTATION

In describing your work to prospective clients, be honest about your work's limits and about any possible negative side effects. Never guarantee results. You can speak of the benefits that you know to be true. For instance, you could say (assuming that it is true to the best of your knowledge) that "many people" have felt calmer, more flexible, more energetic, and so forth after having a massage or a certain kind of bodywork. You can state that "many people" have experienced alleviation of general symptoms. But be aware of the dangers of even subtly leading clients to expect specific cures or fixes. The causes of physical problems are complex, and the outcome of treatments can't be predicted. A colleague says:

> Any time I've done an oversell about the benefits of my method of bodywork, it comes back to haunt me. My reasons are usually well intentioned. Sometimes I'm tempted to do a "hard sell" because I really like a prospective client and *want* to be able to help him. I believe strongly in my work, and sometimes that makes me promise too much. I think it always backfires on me. That will be the client who doesn't get any relief from the treatment.

Scope of Practice

THE ETHICAL STANDARD

Exceeding our **scope of practice** is unethical and often dangerous to our clients. It is unethical to represent ourselves as having training or expertise that we do not possess, such as suggesting that we are skilled in handling serious medical conditions.

We have an obligation to refer clients to appropriately trained professionals and, with the client's permission, to consult with the other professionals who are treating our clients. If we have a client who is ill and currently receiving medical treatment for a serious problem, we should consult with the primary practitioner (with the client's permission) before beginning to work with the client.

IMPLEMENTATION

Practitioners who exceed the scope of their practice are a cause of concern for their colleagues because they reflect poorly on the profession. Some bodyworkers claim to work with emotional and psychological issues, although they have had no training or supervision in these areas. Some bodyworkers claim to have the skills to perform a complex manual technique with only limited training in it. One weekend workshop (or even a few) doesn't make one an expert in physical manipulations—cranial work, visceral manipulation, or whatever is currently the popular practice. It's unethical to advertise ourselves, either on our business cards or verbally, as proficient in a method for which we have only a superficial knowledge or training.

We need to respect the time and training it takes to become a psychotherapist, cranial osteopath, medical doctor, chiropractor, and so forth. At the same time, we need to respect the value of our own skills. Dianne Polseno, ethics columnist for the *Massage Therapy Journal*, says of massage therapy and bodywork, "We are better at what we do than any other health care professional. Other professionals say, 'Tell us what your hands feel.' That's the gift we bring—what we feel under our hands."

If we appreciate the strength and value of our own work, we won't feel the need to pad our resumes.

Another of our unique gifts as health care professionals is the amount of time we spend with our clients and the level of attention and care we give them. There is plenty of healing in simply being with people in a conscious, attentive way—listening to them, listening to their bodies. If we appreciate the strength and value of our own work, we won't feel the need to pad our resumes.

Informed Consent

THE ETHICAL STANDARD

We need to have clients' **informed consent** for (1) the basic treatment or kind of manual therapy that we offer, (2) any work that is near clients' genitals or anus or a woman's breasts, (3) any work that is near an area that we know to be sensitive or triggering for a particular client, and (4) any work that is different from the work we have contracted to do or that the client expects from us.

This means that clients are aware of both the possible benefits and the possible side effects of our work. For instance, they may need to be told that when the body is healing naturally, sometimes clients feel worse before they feel better. Clients also need to know the reasons for a specific treatment or why we need to work in a sensitive area. In addition, they need to be capable of understanding our explanations at the time—they cannot be deeply in an altered state, for instance.

IMPLEMENTATION

Some practitioners obtain written consent from new clients before they begin work. They use a form that explains what the general benefits of the work are, assures clients that there are no guarantees, and states that no medical treatment or diagnosis is involved. Having a client sign such a form also is excellent protection for practitioners. Although it isn't a legal document, it can be a deterrent to lawsuits.

In an intake interview, clients should also be told, either in writing or verbally, about any contraindications to the type of work you do. As you are working, explain and get agreement for any work that is potentially threatening, such as work near the genitals. If you decide to use a different method than what has been agreed upon, explain the method and get the client's consent.

A key to the idea of consent is the understanding that because of transference, clients are not as free to say no as they would ordinarily be. This is especially true if they are already on the table. For this reason, it's best to get clients' consent for new methods before sessions begin and to be clear with clients that they can ask you to stop or can refuse a treatment at any time. If you have an urge to try something different after the session is under way, find a way to ask permission that isn't disruptive and that as much as possible allows the client to refuse.

A friend relates:

> In the middle of a session with a massage therapist I had seen before, I was jolted out of my relaxed state by the lawn mower noise and teeth-rattling pressure of a large electric massager on my back. The massage therapist had never used it before, so it was an unpleasant surprise. I suffered in silence for a while and finally asked him to please stop. He said, "Oh, sorry, I couldn't remember if I'd used this on you before." I didn't say anything, but I was thinking, "So, why didn't you ask me?"

That therapist could have said, "Some clients like for me to use an electric percussive massager on their backs because of the strength of it. Others find it to be too much. It's fine with me if you don't want me to use it. Would you like to try it?" (And the massage therapist could have noted in the client's records whether electric massagers were part of her treatment.)

Disrespect of Other Professionals

THE ETHICAL STANDARD

It's unethical to imply that our skill level or our method of manual therapy is superior to either another practitioner's or another kind of bodywork.

IMPLEMENTATION

We all have ex-clients who think we're skilled and compassionate and those who do not. Take care with another practitioner's reputation.

If you malign another practitioner, it could make you look insecure in your client's eyes. Also, if you make critical remarks about a practitioner your client is seeing or has seen, you are not only questioning that practitioner's competence, but you are also questioning the client's judgment. You want to avoid careless talk, gossip, personal remarks, and assessments about the skills of another practitioner. We all have ex-clients who think we're skilled and compassionate and those who do not. Take care with another practitioner's reputation.

The same goes for maligning other kinds of manual therapies or alternative health practices or being disrespectful of the medical profession. Doing so would make you look small and could offend clients who are loyal to that kind of treatment.

If a client speaks negatively about another practitioner, you need to stay objective. Either remain silent or make a comment related to the client's feelings, such as, "It sounds as if it was an uncomfortable experience for you." You might also ask the client if he thinks his feelings about the previous practitioner could interfere with his ability to enjoy your work. If so, you can suggest that he find a way to get closure with the other practitioner. You can say, "I can't comment about another practitioner's work, but I see that you are still upset and it might be useful to both you and the practitioner if you would write or call him and let him know why you were dissatisfied."

Staying Out of Trouble

Lawsuits and Ethics Complaints

The more you stay inside professional framework and boundaries and the more you honor the therapeutic relationship, the less likely you are to get into serious trouble.

Ethics and the perception of what is ethical are not determined by impersonal rules. They are grounded in your relationship with your clients. In general, if you violate a rule of ethics, you cross a boundary—you go outside the safety of the professional relationship. The more you stay inside professional framework and boundaries and the more you honor the therapeutic relationship, the less likely you are to get into serious trouble.

Lawsuits, Ethics Complaints, and the Therapeutic Relationship

Many ethics complaints and lawsuits against practitioners have little to do with the practitioners' technical skills and a good deal to do with whether the practitioners appear to care about their clients.

A study published in a medical journal showed that a doctor was more likely to be sued if patients felt the doctor was rushing visits, not answering questions, or being rude in some other way. A comparison between doctors who had often been sued and those who hadn't showed no difference in the level of competence of the two groups as perceived by their colleagues. However, the ones who had never been sued were more likely to be seen by their patients as concerned, accessible, and willing to communicate.[1]

Practitioners need to respond in a professional, caring manner to clients who have complaints. Sometimes practitioners make the mistake of stonewalling these clients—not returning their calls or refusing to talk with them. Failing to respond to disappointed or angry clients usually makes things worse. Aside from being an unethical way to handle clients' grievances, this type of behavior usually makes clients angrier, sometimes to the point of filing an ethics complaint. Also, if you do not listen to clients with grievances, you deny yourself the opportunity to learn from clients' feedback.

An administrator for a bodywork school who handles complaints against its graduates agrees that practitioners need to be accessible and open. She says that quite often bodyworkers could avoid having complaints lodged against them if they would simply answer clients' phone calls and allow grievances to be aired. Clients have to be upset or angry in order to file a complaint. In many cases, practitioners who are complained against have followed normal ethical standards but have angered clients by seeming indifferent to their feelings or by emotionally abandoning them in some way. Unless clients are abusive or harassing, the best thing you can do, even if you feel you committed no error, is allow them to speak their minds and let them know that you regret their dissatisfaction.

Framework Exceptions: A Red Flag

Practitioners who have made mistakes or have been complained against have usually had a pattern of making small boundary errors in general or

---

[1]Hickson GB, Federspiel CF, Pichert JW, Miller CS, Gauld-Jaeger J, Bost P. Patient complaints and malpractice risk. JAMA 2002;287(22):3003–3005.

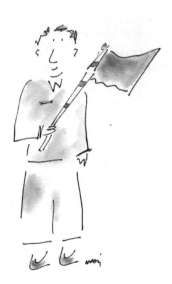

have been careless about boundaries with one particular client. It should be a red flag for you when you're tempted to go outside your own standard policies or the standard practices in your community.

A colleague reports:

> A new client wanted me to give her a discount simply because she said she couldn't afford my prices, although she was working and appeared to be driving a new car. I don't usually give discounts except to those who are physically not able to work, so I refused her at first but eventually gave in because she was so insistent. What a mistake! She turned out to be constantly demanding and complaining, and I never felt that she was satisfied with the work. Although I offered to refer her to another practitioner, she stayed with me through several sessions, complaining all the while. After she stopped coming to me, she filed a complaint with my professional association, saying that my work wasn't useful to her and that I had knowingly cheated her. I found out too late that she had had this same pattern with other kinds of practitioners in the area.

When There Are No Warning Signs: The Need for Documentation and Professional Association

There are instances of practitioners being sued or complained against when there were no significant warning signs.[2] Two things saved them in court: they had carefully documented the client's presenting problems and course of treatment, and they had the backing of a professional association. You need to keep careful notes, especially when you feel uneasy about a client, when you work with clients with medical issues, and when you work with clients who have been abused. But since you never know which client may end up unhappy with your services, it makes sense to keep careful records on all clients. The importance of documentation cannot be stressed enough.

Belonging to a recognized and respected professional group is also helpful. Clients' attorneys will want to make a manual therapy practitioner look sinister, dishonest, or fly-by-night. Belonging to a respected national group enhances practitioners' image. In addition, professional associations often provide witnesses to back up the legitimacy of their methods.

The Right Thing

What's right may vary depending on the client and the situation. How strictly do we interpret the guideline, for instance, that it's not ethical to benefit personally from a client? No one is going to haul us into court if we have cleverly placed our dying ficus plant in the middle of the room, hoping our

---

[2]Individual circumstances of ethics complaints vary. Practitioners who have been officially complained magainst or threatened with a lawsuit should consult an attorney and work with the ethics boards of their organizations.

next client, a regular of many years and owner of a plant shop, will notice it and give us good advice. If the plant shop owner was a new client and we met him at the door with a barrage of questions about our ailing flora, again, we probably wouldn't be sued, but we might lose him as a client or at least make him uneasy.

However, if we use our influence with a regular client to get him to invest in our plant business, we could end up in court with that client if the business fails (or even if it doesn't). To stay out of trouble and avoid taking advantage of our clients, we need a solid understanding of relationship dynamics and the rules of ethics that our profession asks us to follow.

The manual therapies are becoming increasingly popular, and respect for the profession is growing along with its popularity. Each new phase of our professional growth gives us opportunities to use our new power and strength in ways that will benefit our clients and enhance the image of the profession.

QUESTIONS FOR REFLECTION

1. Everyone has some kind of prejudice; your goal is to be aware of what yours are. Think about the ways that you prejudge people based on their appearance, skin color, clothes, or what you think their beliefs to be. Are any of your judgments so severe that you would not want to work with a particular group of people? What can you do to become more understanding of that group?

2. Has a professional ever violated your confidentiality in a small way, for instance, by letting someone else know that you are his client or that you enjoyed a session? How did that feel to you? Has a professional ever told you something about a client that violated the client's confidentiality? Did that influence the way you felt about the practitioner's professionalism? In what way?

3. Have you ever used the services of a professional (massage therapist, bodyworker, chiropractor, physician, or so forth) or any kind of service person (plumber, carpenter) who claimed to know more than he or she really did or who claimed to be able to help you in ways that he or she couldn't? What did you learn from that experience?

4. Have you ever been to a professional who bad-mouthed another professional or said that his own work was superior to that of other professional? What did you learn from that experience?

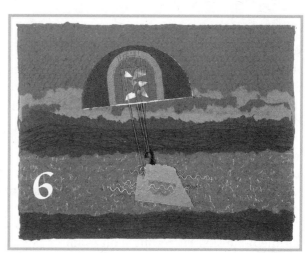

Chapter 6

*B*OUNDARIES AND THE POWER OF WORDS

We communicate with clients in more than words; everything we do speaks volumes to our clients about our professional attitudes and values. Clean, warm offices and a welcoming smile say one thing, and the absence of them says another. The way we touch can communicate, "I'm so interested in working with you and helping you" or "Here's just another bunch of tight muscles."

There is a constant conversation between practitioner and client—much of it nonverbal—about the basic questions of intention and role: "What are the two of us doing in this room together?" This chapter is about the verbal side of that conversation: what do we say to clients, and how do we understand what they are saying to us?

The Power of Our Words

Two powerful influences give our words to clients more weight than they would ordinarily have:

- **Transference:** As explained in Chapter 4, clients are likely to see us as more powerful than they are and perhaps unconsciously relate to us as they do other authority figures in their lives.

- **Altered state:** During sessions, clients are more open than usual, less defended, and closer to their unconscious minds; our words can sink in more deeply.

Because of these two influences, clients may have a heightened sensitivity to what we say. During sessions, clients may see us as an authority or parent figure and be more affected by our words than they ordinarily would

Altered state:
A state of consciousness in which we are more deeply relaxed, less aware of our thinking minds, and more open and vulnerable than we are in our day-to-day functioning.

be. They may, for instance, hear us as being critical when that is not our intention. Our words can be deflating to a client if they sound negative or judgmental. Here's an example of a client's reaction:

> I'm never going back to that massage therapist. He made me feel fat and unattractive. While he was working near my stomach, he said, "I'm sure you're aware of the unhealthy effects of being overweight."

Compassionate words can have an equally strong effect:

> When my bodyworker said, "I know you've had a rough week. I hope I can be helpful to you," I felt myself relax before she even touched me.

Our words can touch clients' hearts or sink their spirits.

Our words can touch clients' hearts or sink their spirits.

Attitudes and Roles

This chapter gives suggestions for useful phrases for common problematic situations with clients. Although we can learn some words to say, no one can hand us a surefire script that will guarantee good results. The words we choose reflect our attitudes about both our clients and our roles. If we understand our roles, the right attitude and the right words will follow.

> A client shows up 15 minutes late. One practitioner says, "You're always late. My time is just as valuable as yours. I wish you would start coming on time. "

> Another says, "We only have 45 minutes left in your hour, but I can help you get rid of lots of knots during that time."

We can hear the difference in their attitudes and in their ideas about their roles. The second practitioner sounds like a professional talking with another adult who needs both education and nurturing. She manages to do two important things at once: set appropriate limits with the underlying message, "You don't get a full hour if you show up late," while showing concern for the client with the underlying message, "I want to help you feel better." She takes care of her professional needs by not letting the client take advantage of her while she also takes care of the client's legitimate needs for help.

The first practitioner starts out sounding like a martyred parent scolding a bad child and then ends up sounding like a whiny child herself. Her statements focus on her own discomfort. She also sounds caught up in countertransference; that is, she seems to be taking the client's lateness personally and forgetting her professional role. Since the clearer we are about our role, the less likely we are to react in a personal way, we need to take another look at our professional role in light of communications.

The Professional Role: Dictator Versus Compassionate Practitioner

To better understand our role, we need to return to the basics of the therapeutic relationship: the concepts of paying attention to the contract, being client-centered, being responsible for a safe environment, and maintaining our own rights. If we don't keep those in mind, we may end up sounding more like little dictators than compassionate professionals.

A common mistake for practitioners (like the first practitioner above) is inadvertently treating clients as if they were wayward children who need to be controlled and ordered around rather than as adults who have come for our professional care and concern. Here are some examples of the "little dictator" attitude:

> Bodyworker Barbara relates, "I'm disgusted with my out-of-shape client who won't do any of the exercises I've given him. I need to tell him that just getting a massage won't help him much if he won't follow up at home."

Aside from being dismayed by Barbara's negative judgment about her client, our concern is whether Barbara has a contract, an agreement with the client to assign him exercises. If the client does not want any service other than a massage, then Barbara is doubly out of bounds, first by deciding what is "best" for him and then by being annoyed when he doesn't do what she thinks he should.

If a practitioner believes she has other services or expertise that would be helpful to the client, she can say, preferably during the initial intake, "You're already helping your health a great deal by coming to get a massage. Just to let you know what else is available, I also offer advice on home exercises (or whatever service) if you are interested."

Since saying even that little might come across as a negative judgment to an out-of-shape client, a better alternative may be to educate clients by spelling out our services in a brochure that we give to clients or by directing clients to our website, if we have one.

> Somatic practitioner Sam says, "My client has such a control problem. She wants to tell me how to do the music, the lighting, even where I can touch her. I tell her that I can't do my best if she won't let me work the way I want to."

We do wonder who has the control problem here. Sam has forgotten that he is responsible for creating an emotionally and physically safe and comfortable environment for the client and that the client's needs are paramount. Certainly, this client has a right to her preferences about music and lighting, within reason, and she has a right to say that she would prefer that the bodyworker not work with some areas of her body.

Suppose a client had a request for where we should or shouldn't work and we think that honoring that request wouldn't serve her well. For instance, he wants us to work so deeply that we are afraid it will cause bruising or injure his tissue. We would then need to educate him: "Although it may seem as if very deep work would help, I can often relieve muscle tension with much less pressure and without the danger of hurting you. Could I try a lighter pressure first?"

Of course, if a client wants us not to work a certain area for reasons of modesty or privacy, we are obligated to honor that request. We may not fully understand the reasons for a client's sensitivities, but we are obligated to comply cheerfully and without taking personal offense.

Communicating With Clients

In light of the basics of the professional relationship, here are general guidelines and suggestions for talking with clients. Of course, you want to find your own style and words.

USE THE CLIENT'S WORDS

When you ask clients during your intake procedure what they want to get from the massage, note how they talk about their bodies, their discomfort, or their lives. Using their own words and images when talking with them will have more impact than using yours.

TALK IN TERMS OF WHAT THE CLIENT'S VALUES ARE

Clients are usually motivated by one of three goals: looking better, feeling better, or performing better—or by some combination of those three. For example, you could tell a ballplayer that if he is less tense, he may be able throw the ball more easily; you could tell a client struggling with illness that lowering stress can help overall health; and you can tell a client concerned about appearance that people often look younger when they are carrying less tension.

TALK TO CLIENTS IN WORDS THEY UNDERSTAND

In particular, you want to avoid New Age jargon if these words are unfamiliar to your audience. For instance, you probably wouldn't tell a banker that you want to release the negative vibrations from his third chakra. You might instead mention that he seems to have a knot in the pit of his stomach.

Talking With Clients During Sessions

Talking with clients who are on the table takes special sensitivity. During the hands-on work, you want to use a different tone of voice or manner than you would use in normal conversation.

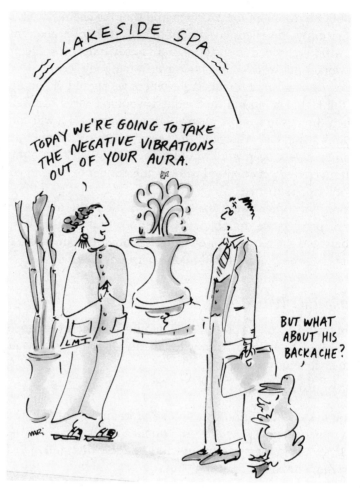

Talk to clients in words they understand.

There are a couple of reasons for this extra care. For one, clients on the table are exposed—although protected by draping, they are often naked. Even if they have their clothes on, they are in a passive position. For another, many people have negative judgments about their bodies. Many clients come to you having been told all their lives by their perhaps well-meaning parents, loved ones, and certainly by the culture that they are too fat or too thin, too flabby, too short, too hairy, and so forth. Unless they are unusually confident, clients may feel some degree of inadequacy, unhappiness, or even shame about their bodies. You don't want to stand there from the safety of being fully clothed and add to their discouragement with careless words. When clients are on the table, the practitioner's words should be reassuring and kind.

Aside from being sensitive to their vulnerability, you also want to provide a space within which clients can turn off their thinking minds and drop into a state of deep relaxation.

In light of those two conditions—wishing to honor clients' vulnerability and allowing a deeply relaxed state—here are some guidelines for talking with clients during the actual session.

SPEAK AS IF TO A PERSON WHO IS ABOUT TO FALL ASLEEP

Use a lighter tone and softer volume than normal conversation. Take care not to say anything that might be upsetting or jarring. Remember that you want to be soothing. If you talk at all, think in terms of using your voice as if it were a third hand.

KEEP YOUR OWN TALKING TO A MINIMUM

Keep in mind that a yakking practitioner is a major complaint of clients. Keep your talking to a minimum and keep it focused on the client. Don't bring up subjects unrelated to the massage.

DON'T ASK QUESTIONS OR TALK IN SUCH A WAY THAT CLIENTS HAVE TO THINK TO RESPOND TO YOU

Even though you want to educate your clients, you don't want to engage peoples' brains with long explanations, speeches, or stories. Don't ask them questions that take thought (except very early on in the session before they are deeply relaxed), such as, "How many times have you hurt this foot?" You don't want to get them involved in left-brain activities, such as counting or analyzing. You can ask them questions that involve the right brain, such as questions about feelings or sensations: "How does this feel?" or "How is this pressure?" Any questions you ask clients who are in an altered state should be no-brainers or, at least, no-left brainers.

KEEP INSTRUCTIONS SIMPLE

To avoid getting people to think, you want to keep instructions simple. For example, some people have trouble distinguishing between right and left, and most people, when they are deeply relaxed, have to think to remember which is which. It can be helpful just to tap lightly on the appropriate side and say, "Would you turn over on this side, please?"

SAY THE OBVIOUS

It's surprising how effective it can be to simply say what seems obvious to you. "You seem to be having a hard time letting go of your right hand. It's been in a fist for much of the session." You don't have to make up fancy explanations or add interpretations. Sometimes just bringing a bodily habit or pattern to a client's awareness makes a big difference.

It's surprising how effective it can be to simply say what seems obvious to you.

USE IMAGES THAT CONVEY THE POSSIBILITY OF CHANGE

You want to let clients know that they can get better, not give the idea they are stuck in an uncomfortable condition. As an example, rather than saying, "This shoulder is like concrete," you can say, "This shoulder joint seems to need more flexibility." Or if an area doesn't have much movement in it, don't say that it looks dead. You can say that it looks "quiet," "asleep," or "as if it wants to move."

FIND SOMETHING POSITIVE TO SAY ABOUT CLIENTS OR ABOUT HOW THEY ARE TAKING CARE OF THEIR BODIES

Compliment your clients for their self-care. They're coming to get a massage or bodywork, aren't they? That's a good start. However, don't comment on how attractive they are. Doing so could sound as if you're sexually interested in them. Speak of "healthy-looking tissue" and legs that "look strong," for example. Just as your positive words can sink in deeper, so can your negative ones. A friend reports:

> I didn't appreciate when a massage therapist told me, "You have the tightest shoulders I've ever seen." That's a title I didn't want to have.

BE CREATIVE WITH IMAGES

Images can help clients stop thinking and let go. Images can touch clients more deeply and stay with the client longer than dry instructions can. For example, you could say, "What if this arm were as loose as a rag doll's?" or "Think of your back as a vast Montana sky." Tailor the images to the client's background and interests.

USE ONLY GENTLE HUMOR

Teasing and sarcasm have a hidden hostility, whereas gentle humor can work well. For instance, to a client with tight shoulders, you could say, "I've been wondering who's been carrying the world around for the rest of us. Looks like it was you."

OF COURSE, NO FLIRTING

Because of the power difference and the client's vulnerability, any flirting can be intrusive or seen as harassing. No matter what your intention or how innocent a remark or tone of voice may seem, flirting with the client sexualizes the situation and is unethical.

TAKE EXTRA CARE WHAT YOU SAY WHEN WORKING AROUND A CLIENT'S HEAD OR FACE

When working around a client's head or face, your words can go even more deeply into their unconscious. Because you're so close to clients' ears that it's easy to sound loud and jarring, it's best not to talk at all. If you do speak, use positive words and images. If you say, for instance, "I want to make your neck looser so you won't have a headache," what may stick in the client's mind is the word "headache." You could say, "It would be great to have more ease here." Or play with images: "See if you can let your neck be as loose as warm taffy."

BE SYMPATHETIC IN YOUR TONE

It's easy for clients to think we're criticizing them. For instance, "You're so tight" can sound like a judgment. We could say instead, "Looks like you've been under some stress."

KEEP THE FOCUS ON THE CLIENT

When a client says, "My husband makes me mad because he won't wash the dishes," you don't need to add, "Oh, mine, too. Isn't it a drag?" Clients are paying for your time and attention, not your life story. Sometimes such a remark would be harmless, and sometimes it could be a problem. Suppose your client is an overworked person who feels that she doesn't get enough personal attention in her life. She may—rightfully—feel intruded on if you take the spotlight away from her.

SUGGEST AND PERSUADE RATHER THAN ORDERING

What could be less relaxing than to have someone order you to "RELAX!"? Instead of that, or commanding, "Let this shoulder go," you could say, "I wonder how it would be if this shoulder could let go."

Dealing With Common Dilemmas

Certain questions and situations come up over and over in our work. Here are some specific ways to handle them, keeping in mind that our goal is to focus on the client's welfare.

Talkative Clients

If a client is talkative, your main concern is whether the talking is good for the client or not. Clients don't have to be totally quiet in order to receive the most benefit from a massage or bodywork. In fact, some clients unwind by talking, especially during the early parts of a massage.

If you see that talking is making a client more tense or getting in the way of his relaxing, then you need to say something. This is an excellent time to educate and suggest rather than order. Rather than saying, "You'll get more out of your massage if you are quiet," you can say, "Notice what happens to your back (shoulders, neck) as you're talking. It's okay for you to talk, but I wonder if it interferes with receiving the full benefit of the work."

Some clients feel obligated to chat, as if the session were a social interaction. Those clients just need reassurance, "If you really want to talk, that's fine, but this is your hour to relax. You don't need to talk if you'd rather be quiet."

> The client was talking so much that it irritated me, so I politely asked her to be quiet.

Is there a polite way to ask a client to shut up? Practitioners really have no right to ask a client to be quiet unless a client is being abusive. Otherwise, clients should be free to sing arias, recite the Gettysburg Address, or talk as much as they want. Your job is to let them know when those activities seem to be getting in the way of their relaxation, not yours.

Sometimes practitioners are distracted by a client's talking because they feel they must respond, as if it were a normal conversation. Actually, all you

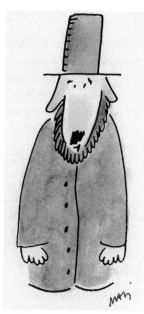

Four score and seven . . .

need to do is say enough to show that you're listening. "Uh huh." . . . "I see." If a client keeps trying to engage you in conversation or if you're newly trained and are having a difficult time focusing, then it's okay to say, "It's fine for you to talk, but if I pay too much attention to talking with you, I can't concentrate on doing a good job."

Clients Who Are Emotional or Want Advice

As clients feel comfortable with you, they sometimes talk about their personal lives or ask for advice. Sometimes as they relax, feelings they've held back in their ordinary lives come up, and they may express their anger or cry. You want to be compassionate with your clients, but when might a response to such expressions be overstepping into a mental health role? Let's sort out when you are being appropriate as a manual therapist and when you might be acting too much like a counselor or psychotherapist.

WHEN CLIENTS WANT ADVICE

When a client is in distress, upset, or having trouble, you may feel that you need to do something about it, to fix it. However, your job isn't to fix your clients' personal lives; your job is to create a safe and relaxing atmosphere for them. You provide a valuable service if you simply listen to your clients.

People who are complaining often don't really want advice; they just want to vent. If that helps them to relax, all you have to do is make sympathetic sounds to show that you're listening and being supportive. "Really?" "That's too bad." Any more than that can be overstepping boundaries.

WHEN CLIENTS ARE EMOTIONAL

Some practitioners are uncomfortable when a client cries; they think they must do something about it or perhaps get the client to stop crying. However, bodywork and massage can bring up held-in feelings, and crying can be a helpful release. When clients cry, you don't need to do anything other than perhaps indicate you're aware of their crying: "Looks like you have a lot of sadness (or feelings) about that." And you might want to offer them a tissue or see if they want you to stop working for a minute. There's no need to do anything else; just your presence can be enough of a comfort.

Some practitioners may go too far interpreting the boundaries between psychotherapy and bodywork. They may think that anything outside of massaging muscles isn't their domain, or they become uncomfortable when a client cries or expresses distress about her personal life. Here's an example of interpreting our role too narrowly:

> My client had just come back from court, where she had officially ended her 20-year marriage. She was very upset, expressing anger at her ex-husband and also crying. I told her that she might need to see a counselor and that I wasn't qualified to help her.

Although there are times when you might need to suggest that a client seek professional counseling, it doesn't take any special training to be a sympathetic ear for clients. If, 6 months after the divorce, this client is still crying and expressing anger at her ex-husband, then you might want to suggest that she seek the services of a counselor. Try to do so in such a way that the client feels supported rather than rejected. "I don't mind your talking about your problems here if it helps you relax, but I wonder if you would also like to see a professional counselor who can support you through this difficult time."

WHEN CLIENTS MAY NEED PROFESSIONAL COUNSELING

In general, you might recommend clients seek professional counseling when they seem unable to come out of normal periods of depression or grief by themselves or when they seem overwhelmed by grief or depression—not just feeling sad or unhappy but unable to engage in their lives or work. Also, if clients seem confused about their lives or unable to cope by themselves or if they often ask you for advice, you should recommend that they seek other help. Again, you want to be compassionate and not sound as if you're rejecting them. You might say, "You seem to have a lot of questions about decisions in your life. I can offer you a sympathetic ear, but I don't have the training to help you sort out your marriage (job, relationships). Have you thought about seeing a counselor?"

If you are unsure about how to work with a client because of his emotional needs, consider getting a consultation from a mental health professional as a valuable resource for yourself.

Certainly, if clients express feelings of wanting to commit suicide, are engaged in self-destructive behavior, or are being harmed by someone else, you must urge them to seek counseling and you should immediately get a consultation yourself from a mental health professional to find out the best way to help this client. Depending on the licensing regulations in your state, you may be required to report a client who is in danger of harming himself or someone else.

Clients Asking Personal Questions

Responding appropriately to a client's personal questions about you can be much more complicated than it looks. Although you may respond spontaneously to questions about yourself from friends or acquaintances, knowing how to respond to clients' questions can take more thought. Often, in order to answer a question well, you'll need to understand the reason the client is asking it.

If you answer a personal question without thought, you could either give out more information than the client needs or than you want to reveal, or your response could shut out the client in an abrupt way. For instance, a male client asking a female practitioner, "Are you married?" could be asking if she could understand the difficulty he is having with his spouse or could be asking if she is available for a date. If you don't know why a client is asking a question and feel uncomfortable with answering, you might say, "I'm curious why you're asking." To be client-centered, you always want to turn the spotlight back on the client—but in a friendly way. You don't want to be abrupt with a client who's just being sociable or trying to connect with you.

If it turns out the client is looking for support for a difficult marital situation, you could say, "I understand how hard it is to keep clear communication with a partner." If you learn the client is looking for a date, you could simply state your policy that you do not socialize with clients.

Clients may ask personal questions for other reasons also. Some clients feel uncomfortable or impolite if the focus of the session is entirely on them. You can let such clients know that they can relax and concentrate only on the work and on their own concerns. And some clients are just curious and friendly and have no hidden motive in asking personal questions.

If there is something dramatic or obvious about you that you know clients will ask about—your foot is in a cast, for instance—have your story ready. You don't want to give each client a 15-minute monologue about how your foot got broken. Again, what you want to discern and respond to is why the client is asking the question. A client inquiring about a practitioner's broken foot could be wondering if the wounded practitioner can now more readily identify with her pain, or she may be asking, "Even though you are injured, can you still help me today?"

Keeping your privacy and keeping the focus on the client can be difficult for those who live in a small town or are part of a community where people know each other's business. However, if a client brings up something they have learned about you from someone else—"How's your bad back/divorce/leaky roof?"—all you need to do is assure them that all is well, that you are fine and ready to give them your attention and best work.

Clients Asking Questions Outside Your Scope of Practice

When clients ask you a question outside your expertise, it's important to be willing to say, "I don't know." It's a respectable answer. You can say, "Sorry, but I don't have any training in that area." Don't pretend to know or try to bluff your way through answering such a question. Not having to know everything can be freeing for you, and your clients will appreciate the honesty of an "I don't know." It educates them about what you do know and what your areas of expertise are. Showing your clients that you honor your limits helps them trust you. Clients won't usually be dismayed or shocked that you don't know everything; they usually just move on to their next concern.

Feeling that you have to know the answer to every question either directly or remotely related to the body can make your work stressful and stifle your curiosity. You could find yourself falling back on rote answers. "The way to work with this kind of knee is to do X." Having to know can make you miss out on what's going on right here, right now, in front of you with this client.

Clients Who Are Demanding

Clients who seem critical, demanding, or controlling can be a challenge; you don't want to take their behavior personally. Avoid getting into negative

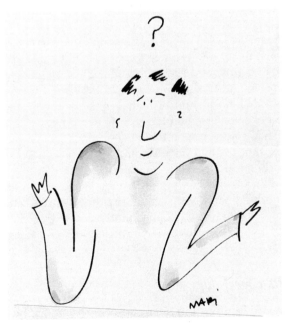

I don't know.

countertransference. Keep in mind that clients may be acting out of fear that stems from past trauma. Although you may never know what clients' histories are, demanding or critical clients are often communicating that it is hard for them to feel safe. Their message may be that they are not sure you are going to pay enough attention to their care. If you respond to their demands with impatience or irritation, you could be proving their assumptions true.

It is better to try to let them know you're doing your best. "Is there anything I can do to make you feel more at ease?" If a client persists in being demanding, you can say gently, "I feel like you're not comfortable, and I want this to be a good experience for you. I hope you will let me know what else I can do." Your honesty and openness may help the client trust that your intentions are good.

It's rare for clients to express directly that they were unsatisfied with your work and that they don't want to work with you again. However, if that happens, it's best to end the relationship in a way that doesn't blame either of you. You could say, "I'm sorry that you're not happy with the massage (or bodywork session). For some reason, we just don't work well together." Or "Perhaps my style of working isn't what you're looking for."

Setting Limits

The ability to set limits gracefully and effectively is vital to our professional lives. Although we may not think of setting limits as a skill that we need to learn, the reality is that our limit-setting skills need to be practiced and polished as much as our hands-on skills.

If we can't set limits well, we can't keep the boundaries safe for ourselves or our clients.

If we can't set limits well, we can't keep the boundaries safe for ourselves or our clients. A colleague reports:

> I had a client who raved about my work and said he was going to tell all his friends about my "miracle work." Well, that kind of praise was hard to take lightly, and I let it interfere with my judgment. When he started coming late and missing appointments without calling, I didn't say anything to him or charge him for the missed time. In fact, I even altered personal plans to create a time slot for him—and he didn't show for the appointment!
>
> I know that I would have set limits sooner with another client, but I was caught up in being "the miracle worker," and that wasn't good for either of us. Every time I didn't set good boundaries, he pushed another limit. I wish I could say that I started setting limits, but the truth is that he just stopped making appointments. I did him a disservice by not being clear about boundaries and expectations.

Setting Limits Gracefully

The most awkward limit-setting dilemmas are how to deal with clients who sexualize the situation and how to maintain boundaries around time and fees. Knowing what to do with clients who make passes or who act sexually inappropriate is discussed in Chapter 8. Here are some ways to make setting limits about time and money easier for you. Of course, you may want to re-phrase these responses in words that feel natural to you.

BE CLEAR ABOUT EXPECTATIONS IN ADVANCE

This is crucial. It's much easier and less awkward to set limits when you know you've been clear with the client about your policies from the begin-ning. It's a good idea to get in the habit of starting to educate clients during the first phone call about your fee policies, time policies, and, if necessary, about the nonsexual nature of your work. For instance, assuming this is your policy, make sure you always say, "If you need to cancel, please let me know at least 24 hours ahead of time so I have time to schedule someone else; otherwise, I'll have to charge you for the session." If you make it a habit, then you don't have to wonder later on whether you've told a client about the policy. About time policies, you can say, "Your appointment will start at 4:00, and that will give us a full hour to work together."

First sessions need to include time not only for gathering information from the client but also for educating the client about your professional standards—in written form, verbal form, or both. That can include policies about late arrival, notice to cancel, payment options (such as whether you take postdated checks), confidentiality, and your right to refuse to work with a client who acts inappropriately. Find policies that you're comfortable with, be clear about them with your clients from the beginning, and then follow through as necessary. Having your policies in writing and asking clients to sign or initial forms is a good idea.

BE CAREFUL ABOUT YOUR TONE

When you have to set a limit, be matter of fact and even sympathetic but not apologetic. "I'm sorry that you couldn't make your appointment last week because you decided to go out of town. Unfortunately, since you didn't let me know you weren't coming in, I have to follow my policy and charge you for that session." Avoid taking a parental or judgmental tone with a client. ("You need to be more considerate of my time.")

SPEAK IN TERMS OF YOUR GENERAL POLICY RATHER THAN PERSONALIZING THE LIMIT

You can depersonalize what you say by referring to your general rules: "It's my policy to charge when a session is cancelled within 24 hours unless the client had an emergency."

PRACTICE WHAT YOU WOULD SAY IN VARIOUS SITUATIONS

Some practitioners have a difficult time setting limits. Remember that set-ting limits is a skill just like learning massage strokes; it takes practice to be-come a pro. To become more comfortable and more effective with limit set-ting, it's a good idea to practice with non-client friends and relatives; try out what you would say in various situations.

Role-playing: Usually a structured exercise in which students or colleagues take a role—for instance, as client or practitioner—and act out a specific situation as a way of becoming more comfortable with handling the situation in real life.

It may sound silly, like play-acting, but **role-playing** is a great way to hone your skills. Even though you may feel mentally prepared to deal with a situation, it helps to say the words out loud. Usually the same feelings that you would have in the actual situation—awkwardness, fear, and so forth—will arise, even though it's not a real-life situation. Also, your colleague can give you useful feedback about the effectiveness of your tone, words, and demeanor.

Here's a success story from Brian Thayer, LMT, a massage therapist, who at the time was a recent graduate of a massage therapy school that uses role-playing. (If you're out of school or your school doesn't offer role-playing, you can set up your own role-playing with willing friends or colleagues.)

> My first paying client turned out to be a great learning experience. I was really nervous beforehand. After the intake process, I left the room to give him privacy, saying, "Please feel free to get undressed to a level that you are comfortable with and get on the table under this sheet face up." When I said "under this sheet," I put my hand under the top sheet and turned it over slightly.
>
> When I returned, I knocked on the door, opened it, and found my client lying face down, completely nude on top of the sheet. As if I wasn't nervous enough!
>
> I took a deep breath and said, "Oops, let me step out of the room while you get under the top sheet and turn face up, please." As I stepped out of the room and closed the door, my calm, centered state escaped me. Taking a deep breath, I knocked on the door again and entered. This time he was under the sheet lying face up, but asked, grabbing the sheet, "Is this really necessary?" My reply was, "Actually, I use proper draping for all my sessions."
>
> I was so pleased that the right words came out of my mouth without a second thought! What made the difference was that I had role-played that very situation with a fellow student, saying what I would say when or if a situation like that came up. They say practice makes perfect: for me, practice made permanent.

Most of us come into this work because we want to help people; an important part of how we help is by setting clear boundaries. Clients feel safer, and practitioners are more at ease when we all know what to expect and where the limits are.

The Right Words

Although our work is centered in the nonverbal, our words make a difference. We want them to enhance our hands-on work and make our jobs easier. Because each client and each situation is unique, there will always be challenges. No matter how long we are in practice, there will always be times when we find ourselves searching for the right words and occasionally stumbling. Our goal is to know that what we say makes a difference and to keep looking for words that connect with our clients.

QUESTIONS FOR REFLECTION

1. You have had two previous sessions with a client. On the day of his third appointment, the weather was fine, but he didn't show up. Practicing with a colleague or friend, put into your own words what you would say or ask when you call this client.

2. Have you ever been a client of a massage therapist or bodyworker who talked in such a way that it was hard for you to stay relaxed? What could that practitioner have done differently to enhance your relaxation?

3. A client calls at the last minute to cancel an appointment because he "just can't get away from work right now." This client cancelled at the last minute once before. At that time, even though you had explained your policy of needing 24 hours notice, you didn't charge him for the missed session. What would you say to him now?

4. Is there a situation involving limit setting that you dread dealing with? How can you make the situation easier for yourself?

5. Imagine you, the practitioner, are a pregnant woman, just starting to show. (You don't have to be pregnant or even a woman to imagine this.) Your client begins to ask you questions about your due date, marital status, and how you feel. How do you keep the conversation client-centered—how to you steer it back to the client? What underlying concerns might the client have about how your pregnancy would affect your professional work and relationship with him or her? How would you find out what those concerns might be, and how would you address them?

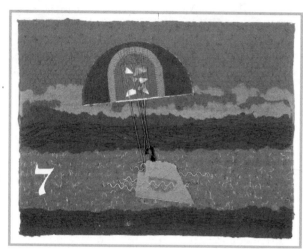

Chapter | 7

SEXUAL BOUNDARIES: PROTECTING OUR CLIENTS

Many of us are led to this work for high-minded reasons. For most, there's a wish to bring greater ease into the lives of others. Some even see this work as a sacred calling, a way to heal the soul and enliven the spirit. But despite the good intentions we bring to our sessions, because we're working closely with the physical body, we can't avoid the murkiness and confusion of sexual issues.

Sometimes clients are sexually attracted to their practitioners. Sometimes practitioners, like any other professionals, are attracted to their clients. The intimacy of our work can be confusing to both client and practitioner. We are touching people, often with a tenderness and gentle attentiveness that is almost like a lover's. When the professional boundaries are clear, it can be wonderfully healing for the client. When they aren't, it can be harmful or even disastrous.

The honest pleasure of sensuality is part of the profession, but the dark possibilities of seduction and exploitation are lurking in the background. How do we keep our sessions safe for our clients and avoid even subtle boundary violations and misunderstandings about sexual boundaries?

The honest pleasure of sensuality is part of the profession, but the dark possibilities of seduction and exploitation are lurking in the background. How do we keep our sessions safe for our clients and avoid even subtle boundary violations and misunderstandings about sexual boundaries?

To begin with, we need to be able to talk honestly with others about these issues. When there isn't enough dialogue, we don't learn from one another. When I started doing research for this book, I was surprised at how complex and painful the stories were from both clients and practitioners. I heard of well-meaning and presumably well-trained practitioners who had stumbled into tangled, destructive situations that might have been avoided had they known the warning signs and acted on them.

- A male massage therapist ends sessions by kissing female clients on the forehead, a seemingly small gesture that could nevertheless be seen as offensive and invasive.
- A female practitioner works close to a client's genitals and is accused of sexual harassment.
- A bodyworker who became sexually involved with a client only later sees how harmful the relationship was to the client.

The emotions in these situations run deep for both client and practitioner. Even if falsely accused of violating a client, a practitioner's distress can be long lasting. And because of the power difference between client and practitioner, the effect on the client when sexual boundaries are crossed, whether intentional or not, can be damaging.

Transference, Countertransference, and Sexual Boundaries

It is in the arena of sexual violations, the most potentially destructive of violations, that we see what a powerful protection professional boundaries can provide. Here's where being sensitive to boundaries and to the effects of transference and countertransference really pays off, steering us clear of harmful mistakes.

The situations described in this chapter present examples of how transference and countertransference can cloud our own judgment and that of our clients.

Positive Transference: Crushes

Sometimes a practitioner is bewildered when a client develops a strong crush on him or her. In Chapter 4, practitioners are warned not to take crushes personally, not to assume that a crush means that the client wants to have a romantic relationship. It's so common for a client to have a crush and so easily misinterpreted that it's worthwhile to explore crushes further: how do they happen and how should we handle them?

It's common for people to develop crushes on any professional who works closely with them, especially when the practitioner is kind to them when they feel vulnerable. For example, female clients often become attached to their divorce lawyers, and patients often idolize compassionate physicians.

We have to keep in mind the special intimacy of a bodywork session. Clients bring all kinds of tender longings, old hurts, and broken hearts to their sessions. And there we are—the picture of kindliness, warmth, and selfless giving. We can seem to be the perfect parent, friend, or confidante they have always wanted. It's easy for clients to "fall in love" with us.

Even though there may be a hint of sexual interest, crushes are usually not the same as grown-up feelings of sexual attraction. These crushes are closer to the kinds of feelings a third grader has for her favorite teacher or the adoration a young boy might have for the star high school athlete.

Here are some suggestions for dealing with crushes so that both client and practitioner are protected.

DON'T TAKE IT PERSONALLY

There's no need to be either dismayed or flattered when a client has an innocent crush on you. You don't want to let your awareness of a client's feelings diminish your warmth and friendliness.

Innocent crushes need to be treated as a sign of the client's trust. The client has judged you to be safe, and you shouldn't make any more of it than that. It can be flattering to have someone wide-eyed over you, hanging on your every word and laughing at your jokes. But you can't let it go to your head. You have to remember that clients have special feelings about you because of the role that you take on, not because of who you are in everyday life. Do your best to remain centered and respectful with clients who have crushes on you.

If a client's attachment to you is upsetting to you, recognize that the problem lies with your discomfort, not the client's feelings (assuming that the client isn't overstepping boundaries). Talk with a trusted teacher or even a mental health counselor to help turn the experience into a healthy learning one for both you and your client.

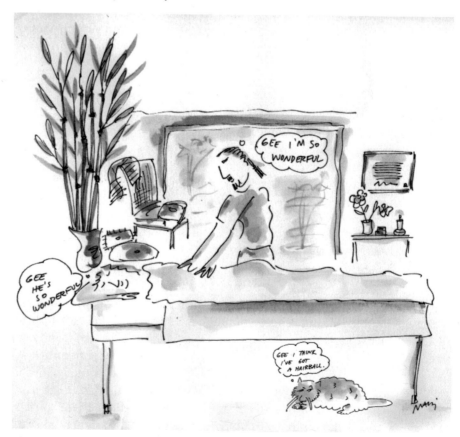

DON'T EMBARRASS THE CLIENT

A colleague reports:

> When I had just graduated from massage therapy school, I was con-
> cerned when one of my clients seemed to have a crush on me. I could
> tell she just adored me. It was kind of flattering, but even though she
> didn't make any suggestions and I knew that she was happily mar-
> ried, it made me uncomfortable. I wasn't sure whether I should talk
> to her about it or not, so I talked to my consultant who helps me with
> problems related to client dynamics. He said not to say anything to
> her and just to keep focusing on giving her a good massage. That was
> good advice. Gradually, the crush seemed to dissipate, and we had a
> solid and warm professional relationship. She was a client for many
> years.

As you can see, there was no need for the practitioner to talk with the
client about her crush. The crush might not have resolved itself so easily if
the client had felt embarrassed or patronized.

PROTECT YOURSELF FROM INAPPROPRIATE CLIENTS

There are times when you do need to protect yourself. Don't assume a crush
is innocent if a client touches you inappropriately, makes a pass at you, or
asks you for a date. You need to set firm limits with such clients. First, make
it clear that such behavior isn't appropriate and that you don't date clients.
Then if you feel comfortable continuing the session or continuing to work
with this client, you may do so. However, if the client seems disrespectful,
you just don't trust him, or you feel uneasy, you can tell him the session is
over and that he's not welcome as a client again.

TAKE CARE WITH BOUNDARIES

Clients who have crushes sometimes invite their practitioners to socialize
with them. What they often want is not the usual give-and-take of a social
relationship but a continuation of the therapeutic relationship in which the
focus is on them. It's not a good idea to see any clients outside the office setting—this is particularly true of clients with crushes. If you're tempted to do
so, be honest with yourself. Are you enjoying the crush? Are you hoping to
flirt or take it further? If a client with a crush on you asked you to a party
and you showed up, couldn't that give the message that you're interested in
the client? You have to respect the vulnerability of your clients by keeping
the relationship within professional boundaries.

Positive Countertransference: "Special" Clients

Feeling that one client is exceptional and different from your other clients,
wanting to rush into dating that client, thinking that others wouldn't understand the "special" feelings the two of you have—all these are warning

signs. Intense feelings about clients are generally indications of counter-transference. When there is that adolescent sense that the intensity of the attraction or the specialness of the relationship between the two of you justifies breaking the rules, it is a red flag.

Of course, all your clients are special and need to be appreciated for their uniqueness. But being overwhelmed with attraction to a client or intensely identifying with a client is different from having compassion for or even loving your clients. A sense of specialness about a client is a problem when it leads you to treat that client differently from others, when you feel that the client is so special that you don't have to adhere to the usual boundaries when working with him or her. In the therapeutic relationship, this can be traumatizing for both parties, as in this story told by a colleague:

> A woman related that during the course of seeing a female body-worker for many months, she developed an intense transference—she was deeply infatuated with her practitioner. She also felt that the practitioner was very drawn to her and that the practitioner had lost her objectivity. The relationship developed into an inappropriate situation in which, under the guise of therapy, the therapist had touched the client's breasts and genitals during several sessions. The client ended up feeling emotionally and physically seduced and damaged. Her confused feelings of shame and guilt were so powerful that she had never discussed this relationship with anyone. She was only able to discuss it in response to an online questionnaire in which she could remain totally anonymous.

No matter how seductive the client or how equal you feel the relationship is, practitioners are responsible for keeping good professional boundaries. It's important to remember that your relationships with clients are never equal and that you can damage your clients if you act on inappropriate feelings. When clients are "in love" with you or have crushes on you, those feelings can be part of a positive therapeutic experience if boundaries are kept. If you are tempted to take the relationship further, get a consultation from a mental health professional to help you sort out your feelings.

Dating an Ex-Client

Given the dynamics of transference and countertransference, you can see the problems with dating an ex-client. Is it ever ethical or safe for the client? The answer is, it depends. It depends on the professional relationship, the intensity of the transference, how emotionally stable the client is, how emotionally stable the practitioner is, and how much time has elapsed since the therapeutic work. The most important question is whether the transference and countertransference feelings are resolved, and that's a complex issue to gauge.

The rules of many manual therapy associations say that it may be okay to date a client if you wait several months after ending the professional relationship, usually 6 months to 1 year. Other professional associations don't approve of such dating no matter how much time has gone by. Practitioners need to check with the licensing laws in their states and the ethical guidelines of their professional organizations.

The reason for delaying social interaction after concluding the therapeutic relationship is to make sure that neither the client nor the practitioner is still caught up in the rosy glow of transference and countertransference. There needs to be time for reality to set in.

Regardless of what the ethical rules allow, however, there may be clients that you could never ethically date. There are some circumstances that would make the transference so strong that a sexual relationship would never be appropriate with the client. For instance, if a client has been helped out of great physical or emotional pain by a practitioner, he or she might always see that practitioner as a larger-than-life hero. A practitioner who is able to provide relief from pain when all other methods have failed may always seem like a savior to that client. Also, any circumstances that would make a client look up to a practitioner may help create a relationship in which there can never be equal power—for instance, if a bodyworker is a teacher or is well known in the community.

However, in some circumstances, dating an ex-client might not bring problems. For example, if a bodyworker in a health spa saw a client once for a sports massage, it is more likely that a strong transference did not develop. Even then, the bodyworker would have to consider how dating an ex-client would affect his reputation and the reputation of the profession.

> A former client with a crush on his bodyworker asked her for a date. Because she was able to honestly say that she never dates ex-clients, he was able to save face and, later, resume his professional relationship with her. Suppose the bodyworker had refused him and he knew of other ex-clients she had dated? Suppose she had accepted, had developed a relationship with him, and it had ended in quarrels?

You also have to consider that if present clients heard that you were dating an ex-client, it might interfere with their therapeutic relationship with you.

Practitioners of **emotionally oriented bodywork** that evokes deep transference should give serious consideration before beginning to date an ex-client. The possibility for taking advantage of a former client's transference is strong.

In any circumstances, you must take into account the emotional stability of the client. For instance, does the client have solid self-esteem, or is she prone to depression, easily influenced, in crisis, or facing any other situation that would make her emotionally fragile? Some clients may never be able to see themselves as equals with their practitioner.

Emotionally oriented bodywork (also called psychologically oriented bodywork): Manual therapy that is based on the idea that physical tension and restriction are related to unconscious patterns of holding that the client has adopted, often early in life, to cope with his or her emotional environment. The practitioner facilitates the client in releasing these holdings for the greater emotional and physical well-being of the client.

Whether to date an ex-client isn't a decision to make lightly. Even if you are certain that you're not taking advantage of a client, just by dating an ex-client you're opening yourself to scrutiny by your colleagues and risking damage to your reputation and that of the profession.

Dual Relationships

You would think that the more someone knows you, the less chance that they would misread your intentions. However, the opposite is often true.

Dual relationships can cause problems with sexual boundaries; in dual relationships, the boundaries are already blurred. Working with people you know in some other way, doing trades, or working with people who share a community with you may sometimes lead to confusion about sexual boundaries. You would think that the more someone knows you, the less chance that they would misread your intentions. However, the opposite is often true. Here's how the dynamic of transference affected a trade between two colleagues:

> Sally, a massage therapist who had been sexually abused by her father, agreed to do a trade with Jim for sessions in his form of psychologically oriented bodywork. As the trade went on, transference factors caused her to unconsciously see Jim as a father figure. At the same time, the bodywork was bringing up memories and feelings about her abuse.
>
> To fulfill her side of the trade, she gave Jim a massage every other week. On a deep level, it was confusing to Sally. It was too hard to relate to Jim as both her therapist and a client whose naked body she was touching. For instance, she began to wonder if Jim was sexually interested in her, even though he seemed happily married. Although she discussed her concerns with Jim and believed him when he said he wasn't attracted to her, she realized she was too uncomfortable with the trade and ended it.

Trades can make it difficult to maintain clear and clean boundaries. Although they can work out well, it usually takes extra effort to make sure they do. Practitioners doing emotionally oriented work or deep structural work should probably never do trades for bodywork. The confusion brought about by transference and countertransference makes such trades potentially harmful.

The same confusion can occur if you are working with someone who is part of a "family" group that you're in—for instance, you're both serious students of the same yoga teacher, you're in the same Buddhist community, or you're members of the same church. When you're working with such a person, you need to be alert to the negative transference about "family" that can get projected onto you because of your mutual association with that group; not everyone has good memories of family. Even though whatever group you both belong to may be spiritual and well intentioned, your client may have buried in his unconscious the idea that "family" means abuse and may associate you with that negative picture.

Secrets

You are headed for trouble any time you are doing something with a client or even having a feeling about a client that you want to keep secret or that you would not share with your colleagues. When you feel that desire for secrecy, the best thing to do is get it out in the open. As hard as it may seem, share your secret with a teacher or consultant. It could be that there is no reason for you to feel uncomfortable. Or it could be that you need help with the client before the situation turns into an even more difficult problem.

Clients Who Have Been Sexually Abused

As we have seen, transference can lead clients to unconsciously associate us with past authority figures. This transference can be especially charged if a client was sexually abused as a child.

When children are sexually abused, the abuser is often a member of the family—perhaps a father, mother, or older relative. Abused children can rightfully feel betrayed: someone who was supposed to be protecting them and taking care of them has taken advantage of them. Sometimes those feelings of betrayal and mistrust linger, usually on an unconscious level, even after the individual becomes an adult. Although it is not true of every individual who was sexually abused, some clients who were abused as children will transfer those feelings of mistrust onto anyone who is a caregiver or authority figure, which can include bodywork practitioners.

Because of these associations, some clients come to sessions with an underlying (and usually unconscious) distrust of the practitioner and perhaps with the expectation that the practitioner will, at the least, not take good care of them and, at the most, exploit them.

Other kinds of behavior may be seen in clients who have been sexually abused. They may be hyper-alert to signs of danger or seduction and, therefore, more likely to misread a careless word or gesture. They may have a distorted sense of what appropriate boundaries are, making them blind to a truly dangerous situation when a therapist is being inappropriate or even causing them to test the intentions of the practitioner by being seductive themselves.

Interactions with sexually abused clients can be complicated if the practitioner has also experienced such abuse. Practitioners who have a history of being abused can have the same kinds of distorted perceptions that clients do. They can assume that a client has sexual intentions when he does not, or they can fail to respond adequately when a client actually is being offensive. Practitioners who have been sexually abused may also be unable to see their own seductiveness or inappropriateness with a client. Boundary violations may unconsciously feel comfortable and familiar to them.

Here are a couple of examples of what can happen:

> Before the session begins, a female massage therapist announces to a new male client who has not shown any signs of acting inappropriately that she has a stun gun that she will use if he gets out of line.

> A male bodyworker flirts with all his female clients and often accepts social invitations from them.

In the first example, the practitioner is being overly self-protective; in the second, the practitioner cannot see the violations he is committing. (Of course, practitioners can overreact or commit violations without having a history of being abused.)

Because of the potential for confusion and missteps, the safest way to avoid making serious errors with clients is to stick to accepted boundaries and provide a stable framework. We may never know what history a client brings to the table, and it is not our place to ask clients whether they have been sexually abused. However, we are safer if we treat all clients with the care that we would use if we knew that they were in need of special sensitivity.

Working With Clients Who Have Been Sexually Abused

Statistics on sexual abuse vary. Some say that at least one in three women and one in twelve men has been sexually abused. Because so many people have experienced sexual abuse that you probably cannot avoid working with someone who has, it is a good idea to be educated about how to work with such clients. Also, if you have a client who is actively dealing with issues of sexual abuse in psychotherapy, you need to contact the client's psychotherapist (with the client's written permission) to make sure that the work you are doing is helpful to the client. Having supervision from that psychotherapist or another mental health professional also is very helpful.

Not every client who has been sexually abused is in need of counseling. However, if you have reason to believe that a client needs to see a psychotherapist—for instance, the client seems depressed or self-destructive—you can suggest counseling. While you may provide your regular massage therapy services to such a client, never attempt to work with sexual abuse issues on your own. Such work takes experience and training. For your own safety—for instance, to avoid being falsely accused of sexual harassment by an overly vigilant client—it's a good idea to seek out outside help with the psychological dynamics of the relationship.

All manual therapists need to educate themselves about working with clients who have been sexually abused by reading relevant literature and attending workshops. On rare occasions, such clients have flashbacks during the session: they experience the memory of the abuse as if it is happening in the moment. Education can prepare you to deal with such situations and can help you feel more confident with other signs of sexual abuse.

Most of the effects of sexual abuse that you will encounter are not dramatic. The signs of abuse that you will see most often are usually less obvious. As noted previously, such clients may be more wary and slow to trust. They may seem controlling or demanding. They may have a more difficult time letting go and relaxing. Or they may be seductive.

There are simple ways that you can help sexually abused clients feel safer. Of course, these precautions are valuable in working with any client.

DON'T PUSH CLIENTS

If clients seem numb in a particular area, don't push them to feel it. Work somewhere else. If a client shares a memory of abuse but doesn't have a complete picture, don't push him or her to remember it. Remembering an incident of abuse isn't necessary to healing, and it can often be re-traumatizing for the client. Leave the treatment of sexual abuse issues to those who have extensive training and experience.

STAY SYMPATHETIC BUT OBJECTIVE

If a client tells you about an experience of being sexually abused, be a sympathetic listener but be careful about sharing your opinion or experience. For instance, talking about what a bad person the perpetrator was is not a good idea. If the perpetrator was also someone the client felt close to, the client may have mixed and confusing feelings about the person, including loyalty or affection.

MAKE SURE CLIENTS HAVE A VOICE

Because of transference and feelings of dependency, clients often don't speak up when you're making them uncomfortable. This is especially true when the discomfort is around a sexual issue. Even if the client is an acquaintance or colleague and even if the person is usually assertive in the outside world, once in the role of client, she or he can have a hard time saying no.

> A successful businesswoman receiving a massage in a spa thought that the practitioner was working too close to her genitals. She didn't think the massage therapist, an older woman, was making sexual advances, but she was still uncomfortable. In the business world, the businesswoman had a diplomatic but straightforward style of dealing with people and gave critical feedback easily. In the role of client, however, she said nothing but never went back to that therapist.

It can help clients voice their feelings if you demonstrate in many ways your interest in hearing how they feel and what they have to say. Bill Scholl, a Trager instructor, says he makes sure to ask clients to let him know if anything he does makes them uncomfortable. He does this even with clients he has worked with many times before. Let clients know that they can always ask you to stop, even if they do not have a reason that seems rational and even if they feel that they are being rude by doing so. Avoid the appearance of dominating a client.

Other Cautions and Red Flags

There are a number of other areas where it makes sense to be cautious and to think of the potential for misinterpretation by a vulnerable client.

Professional Appearance

Short shorts, tank tops, and cleavage are for off-hours. Don't dress as if you're going out on a date or to the beach. You can be comfortable and still look like a reliable professional. Basically, you want to wear clean, neat, loose clothes that don't draw attention to your body.

In most parts of the country, visible tattoos and unusual facial rings, such as nose or eyebrow rings, raise other people's eyebrows and make you have to work harder to convince them that you are safe and professional. Let your work show people how special you are—not your jewelry or body art.

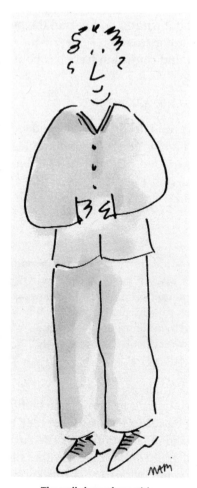

The well-dressed practitioner.

Language

You need to be careful that your language isn't even remotely suggestive or flirtatious. For instance, it's best not to tell clients, "Take off your clothes." That sounds like an order, and it is too close to words that would be used in a sexual encounter. Instead, say something such as, "I'll leave the room so that you can get ready for the session."

Choose your words carefully when you say anything about a client's body. Even saying "Why do you criticize your body? You look great!" can sound overly personal or suggestive. You might sometimes want to compliment a client who seems to have a negative body image. When clients make unflattering comments about their bodies, you can say something general such as, "Gosh, women (or just people) are so hard on themselves about how they look." To be sure you avoid being heard as expressing sexual attraction, however, you're better off avoiding all comments about how you think the client's body looks aesthetically. Besides having the potential to be seen as a come-on, making such a remark puts you in the position of being an expert on how bodies should look, which, of course, you're not.

Draping

Draping is always a good idea. In most massage licensing, it is the law. For deep work or emotional work, having the client wear underpants or briefs in addition to draping is a must. When in doubt, go for more cover rather than for less. It's respectful to the client's privacy and a way to protect yourself from misunderstandings.

Disrobing

Clients need to dress and undress in private, and they need to know that they do not have to undress at all if it makes them uncomfortable. Let them know that they can wear a bathing suit or whatever else is suitable—for instance, athletic shorts and a comfortable bra or tank top. If necessary, you can explain how it will limit your ability to work with them if they choose to leave clothes on, but always make sure they know it is their decision.

Locked Doors

The question of whether or not the door was locked has been a crucial point in some court cases in which a practitioner was sued for sexual harassment. Even if a client isn't locked in or could unlock the door, the point has been raised that the client should be able to leave the room quickly and easily. In many situations, a practitioner may want to lock the door to protect the client from unwanted intrusion, such as a stranger wandering into an office by mistake. A cautious way to handle that type of situation is to explain your reasons for wanting to lock the door and give clients the option of it being locked or unlocked.

Intrusive Work

Some manual therapies can involve intrusive work. If you have good reason to work in an area near a client's genitals, near the coccyx, or near a woman's breasts, you can tell the client in a matter-of-fact way what you are about to do and why. Use terms they can understand—breastbone or tailbone, for instance, instead of sternum or coccyx. "It might be a good idea to work on the muscles around your tailbone because it could be useful to free them up. However, if that makes you uncomfortable, it's fine to skip that area." Let clients decide if it's all right. Watch to see if it really is okay or whether they tense up or seem to be trying to act as if it's fine when it really isn't. The safest plan is to let clients know before the session begins that the session might involve intrusive work and get their consent before they are in the more vulnerable state of being on the table. In some parts of Canada, practitioners are required to get prior consent in writing for such work.

Cautious behavior protects both you and your clients. In the altered state that clients enter into, they can get confused about both your intentions and where your hands actually are. Bring those things into their conscious awareness by giving clients specifics.

You may not know what areas are sensitive for a particular client. Heida Brenneke of the Brenneke School of Massage in Seattle makes this point: "Massage therapists think too narrowly about where a memory of sexual abuse may be in the body—if, for instance, someone was pinned down by her shoulders during abuse, working in that area could bring up the memory." Any of your work has the potential to trigger a memory of sexual abuse. Therefore, you always want to keep an eye out for signs of discomfort from the client, such as their becoming more tense or numb.

Expressions of Affection

Although it may come from genuine caring, initiating hugs with clients isn't a good idea. Mandatory hugs can be very intrusive for clients. The same is true, only more so, for kissing on the forehead or cheek. We may think that clients would welcome any expressions of affection. "But love heals—why not hugs?" goes the argument that Lucy Liben of the Swedish Institute in New York hears from some students. Actually, understanding is what heals. And that may involve your understanding that, for some clients, being in charge of their own personal space is healing. As the client is leaving the session, you can show through your body language that you are available for a hug if the client wants to initiate one (assuming that you are) without forcing the issue. Giving clients the choice is another way to respect their boundaries.

Unintentional Touching

When asked about uncomfortable experiences, clients often cite situations in which some part of a practitioner's body other than hands touched them or the practitioner leaned against them. This is usually accidental on the part of the practitioner, but it can be disturbing to the client. One woman reports:

> In the middle of a massage from a male practitioner, he leaned against my hip with his belly to reach the other side of me, instead of walking around the table. I was so uncomfortable that I had a difficult time relaxing for the rest of the session, wondering whether there would be another incident.

Not every client will react strongly to unintentional or careless touching. However, some will. You do not want to prop yourself against clients as if they were furniture. Of course, if your technique requires you to touch clients with other parts of your body or to lean against them, the reasons for this intrusiveness should be explained to clients, and their consent must be given.

You also want to be careful about wearing sleeves that dangle and things that could brush against clients. In the open and receptive state induced by bodywork, clients shouldn't have to figure out what is touching them.

The Power of Touch

We cannot ignore sexual issues when learning to work with our clients. Because the sensuality of healing touch that we offer is often so close to the sensuality of sex, we need to be all the more careful to maintain clear sexual boundaries with clients. The manual therapies are intimate and can bring up issues about sexuality, both for us and for our clients.

This work can be a blessing for people who are starved for safe and respectful touch. However, we're always skating the edge between the sacred and the profane. It speaks to the goodwill and compassion of practitioners that we so often succeed in keeping the balance on the side of the sacred.

QUESTIONS FOR REFLECTION

1. Has a manual therapy practitioner or other health care provider ever said or done something that felt like a violation of your sexual boundaries or that made you uncomfortable? Did you say something to the practitioner, either at the time or later? Did you tell anyone? If this has not happened to you, have you heard of such an incident happening to a friend or colleague? What feelings did that person have about the incident?

2. Have you ever looked up to or had a crush on a practitioner of any kind who worked closely with you? Do you feel that it would have been appropriate if the practitioner had entered into a romantic relationship with you? Why or why not?

3. Is there anything in your history that might help you be more sensitive to issues of sexual boundaries with clients? Is there anything that might get in the way of your being comfortable with setting clear sexual boundaries with clients?

4. Imagine that you're single and run into an ex-client (also single) at a party. There seems to be a mutual attraction that you weren't aware of while you were working with the client. You are thinking of asking this person for a date. As a professional, what concerns would you have in evaluating whether it would be ethical or wise to do so?

5. Have you ever had a professional massage in which the draping wasn't adequate? Were you uncomfortable because of it? If you weren't, could you imagine circumstances in which you would be?

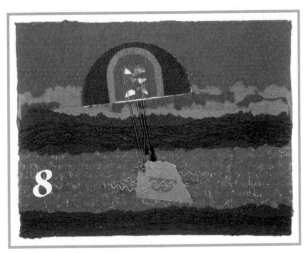

Chapter 8

*S*EXUAL BOUNDARIES: PROTECTING OURSELVES

We live in a culture in which massage is sometimes associated with sex. Many people are uneducated about the manual therapies and do not appreciate that we are professionals who work with therapeutic intention. It's distressing but understandable that some of the public might still think that all massage practitioners offer sexual services. How often have we seen massage therapists portrayed in television sitcoms or movies as crossing the line? How often have new acquaintances made sexual innuendoes and jokes about our work? To complicate matters, those who do offer sexual services often bill themselves as practicing massage. The intimacy of our work leaves us open to misunderstandings and false accusations.

Protecting Yourself From the Public's Misunderstanding

Unfortunately, the accusations aren't always false. Somatic practitioners do sometimes cross ethical boundaries about sexual behavior—probably no more than other professionals do, but our profession is particularly vulnerable to being linked with sex. When other practitioners violate sexual boundaries, it can damage not only their own reputations but also those of the professionals in their community. How do we protect ourselves from potential confusion and harm, both from the public and from within our ranks?

Mistaken Identity

If you advertise your massage or bodywork practice publicly, you may not be able to avoid the occasional low moment of someone assuming that you are offering sexual services. Unless you choose your clientele carefully, you have to be prepared for the occasional inappropriate or offensive questions on the phone and perhaps even in your office. Here's an example:

> A colleague was befuddled when a first-time client asked if she provided "a happy ending." Not having heard this euphemism for sexual release, she said, "Oh, yes, I like my clients to enjoy their massages." When he then described what he wanted in plainer language, she was quick to tell him she didn't offer sexual services and that she wouldn't work with him if that was what he wanted.

While fielding such questions on the phone can be uncomfortable, dealing in person with a client who expects sex can be annoying and even frightening. Although it's only a remote possibility, this situation could also be dangerous.

Some female practitioners avoid these problems altogether by limiting their practice to female clients. (Women clients are generally less sexually aggressive than men. They can be seductive, for instance, but aren't as likely either to expect sexual services or ask for them.) Some practitioners don't work with anyone who hasn't been referred by someone they trust. Regardless of your gender, if you advertise or post your business card in a public place, there may be no foolproof way to avoid such interactions, but there are ways you can lessen their frequency and protect yourself.

Advertising and Business Cards

Be careful when you advertise in a publication. Find out where your ad will be placed. Will it run next to the ads in which "massage" is a code word for sex? Will it show up next to ads for places with dubious names such as Buffy's Massage and Pleasure Spa? If so, you might want to reconsider advertising in that publication.

It's also helpful to consider the nature of a publication's readership. If you live in a big city, running an ad in a smaller, weekly, more trendy newspaper is usually safer than using the daily newspaper or the Yellow Pages. Readers of the smaller papers are often more attuned to alternative health practices. Wherever you advertise, it's also a good idea to avoid the words "release," "total relaxation," and "full-body massage." These phrases can sound like veiled sexual references. Avoid them, too, when you're on the phone with prospective clients.

Make sure your business card doesn't send a mixed message. Cards that give no last name, that simply say, "Massage by Bill" or "Relaxing Massage by Jennifer" are less professional and may give clients the impression you have something to hide. Since sex workers usually don't give their last names when they advertise, it's important that you provide your full name and credentials (professional association membership, state license number, and so forth) to establish that you're a legitimate massage therapist. Using the term "therapeutic massage" and naming your particular technique, such as sports massage, are also helpful. To ensure your privacy and professionalism, list your business number, not your personal one.

Since sex workers aren't likely to go to the trouble of setting up a legitimate-looking website, having a website and listing it in your advertising also helps establish your work as nonsexual.

Screening Clients by Phone

Clients who are looking for more than just a massage may not always say so in the initial phone call. Before the prevalence of cell phones, it was easier to figure out which prospective clients wanted something else. When I first started out as a massage therapist, there was a type of call that I named "the dreaded phone booth call." When I could hear traffic in the background, I always said I wasn't in. The traffic noise told me that these people were calling from a phone booth, and it seemed too likely that the callers were avoiding calling from their home or office because they thought they were doing something illicit.

Since almost everyone uses cell phones these days, the sound of traffic noise is not unusual anymore; however, there are other red flags that signal the wrong kind of call. If people call on Friday afternoon around 5:00, they may be more likely to be facing a weekend alone and looking for "companionship." Such callers often don't want to make an appointment unless you can see them immediately, within an hour or two. Also, look out for callers who initially don't give their full name or who give no name at all.

Here are some other ways to screen out clients who are calling for the wrong reason.

ASK FOR INFORMATION

Ask for callers' full names and callback numbers. If they refuse, don't make the appointment. Also, you can ask about their previous experience with massage. If they've been to a massage therapist you know is legitimate or if they seem to be familiar with professional bodywork, that's a good sign.

CLARIFY YOUR BOUNDARIES

When in doubt, you can say, "I like to make it clear to all new clients that I offer only a nonsexual, therapeutic massage." This is not always convincing, however, because sex workers who call themselves masseuses will say the same thing in case the caller is from the vice squad.

TRUST YOUR INTUITION

If you have an uneasy feeling about someone, don't make the appointment. It is better to lose a session fee than to put yourself in danger.

If you have an uneasy feeling about someone, don't make the appointment.

Staying Safe During the Session

Usually, the worst a client interested in sexual services does is injure your professional dignity and pride. However, in rare cases, massage therapists have been assaulted by such clients. As long as there's even a slight danger, there's no need to take risks. Here are some ways to stay safe.

WORK IN A SAFE SETTING

Working in an office building is usually safer and appears more professional to prospective clients than working out of your home. Leading a client through your home to where the bedrooms are (and your office now is) can be suggestive to new clients.

Don't work in an isolated office with clients you don't know. Don't schedule new clients late in the day or at times when no one else is around.

BE ESPECIALLY CAREFUL ABOUT OUTCALLS

Outcalls require you to go into someone else's home and be at the mercy of any hidden agendas the client might have. Screen such calls carefully or only do outcalls with people who have been referred by someone you trust.

> One male massage therapist related a story of being set up by a female client who wanted to make her boyfriend jealous. During the outcall, the client threw the draping off her chest just as her boyfriend burst through the door. The boyfriend made angry accusations, and the massage therapist fled, unharmed but wiser.

SPELL OUT YOUR POLICIES IN WRITING

As part of their intake process, some massage therapists ask new clients to sign an agreement stating that the practitioner has the right to terminate a session if the client speaks or acts inappropriately. The clearer you can make it from the beginning that this is a nonsexual massage, the easier it will be for you to avoid inappropriate requests.

CHOOSE YOUR EMPLOYERS WELL

Before working at a spa, for instance, make sure your employer will back you up if you choose to end a session or choose not to work with a client who has made sexual requests.

Educating Clients

There is no set way to respond when a client on the table asks you for something that is inappropriate. It depends on your own comfort level, how safe the setting is, and your history with the client. Some clients are simply misinformed; sometimes all you have to do is educate them and set limits.

When a client misunderstands, you don't need to waste your energy on a fit of righteous indignation. There's no need to take it personally. Here's a great example of how one massage therapist handled an awkward situation. The story was told by Lee Phillips, a massage therapist in Levittown, Pennsylvania:

A man called and made an appointment. He showed up on time and looked around the room, which was clean and airy with a massage table in the middle, anatomy posters on the walls, and books in the bookshelf. The massage therapist was dressed in her usual style of a polo shirt and long pants. Seeing the man's perplexed expression, she said "This isn't what you were expecting, is it?"

"Er . . . uh . . .no," he mumbled.

"Then I'll get a phone book for you if you'd like. You may use my phone, " the massage therapist said.

"Uh . . . thanks."

She gave him the Yellow Pages, open to "Massage—Other" (which was next to "Massage—Therapeutic") and left the room. Shortly, he came out, said, "Thank you," and quickly left.

Setting Limits

If a client makes an inappropriate sexual suggestion during the session, you should respond to it immediately:

- Stop the massage.
- Take your hands off the client's body.
- Address the situation.
- Define your boundaries.

You can say, "I want to make it clear that this is a nonsexual massage and I won't work with anyone who is acting inappropriately." Many practitioners, especially if the client is physically stimulating himself, would simply end the massage then and leave the room, regardless of what the client says. Others, depending on their comfort level, might give a client who has made an inappropriate remark a chance to improve his behavior. Sometimes a client doesn't intend to be offensive; he just doesn't know better.

If you're not sure what the client's intentions are but still feel uncomfortable or threatened by his comments or behavior, trust your feelings and end the session. You can say, "Perhaps you don't mean any harm, but I'm not comfortable working with you any more. I'll wait outside while you get dressed."

Most massage therapists are so grateful when these clients leave that they don't ask for payment. (Others get payment at the start of a session.) Technically, clients may owe the fee for a massage or half a massage, but it's up to you whether to make an issue of it.

Self-Presentation

If you're getting a high percentage of calls or office encounters in which the clients think you're offering sex, you need to take a look at how you're presenting yourself. This could be as simple as changing your ads or how you dress or as complicated as looking at what your intentions really are. You might need to get another perspective—you could ask a mentor or more experienced practitioner for honest feedback.

Perhaps the day will come that when people think of massage, they think only of its many health benefits and the boost it gives to both physical and emotional well-being. Until that time, clear communication in all stages of our contacts with clients can help educate those who need it and protect us from misunderstandings.

The Erection Dilemma: Protecting Both Ourselves and Our Clients

How should a practitioner respond when a client has an erection during the session? Again, it depends on the situation, the client, and your comfort level. Some practitioners wrongly believe that if a man is having an erection, the practitioner must immediately end the massage. There is the misconception that for a man to have an erection, he must be deliberately sexualizing the situation and either mentally or physically stimulating himself. However, the truth is that having an erection can be an innocent accident and just as embarrassing to the client as it may be anxiety producing for the practitioner.

Erections can occur as a natural physiological response to being touched. One of my teachers in massage school described them as being

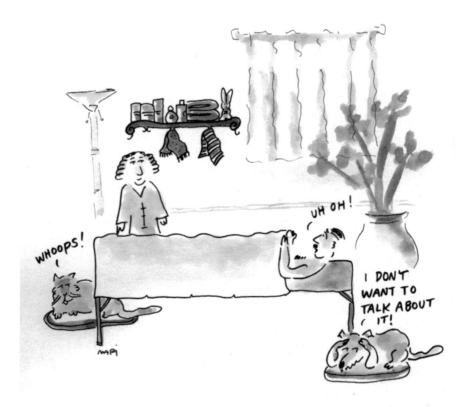

"like a dog wagging his tail"—an automatic physiological response to pleasure. Men report that they can be floating along enjoying the sensuality of a massage without any sexual thoughts or feelings of attraction to the therapist, and then . . . oops, their enjoyment has become visible. Younger men can have erections, as one therapist put it, "if the wind changes direction" and certainly from the intimacy of a massage.

When an erection occurs, it can make both the client and the practitioner feel vulnerable. If you respond with unnecessary disapproval and fear, it's a disservice to an already embarrassed client. Yet you have to guard against the threat of a disrespectful, abusive client. It's a tricky situation.

Aside from the misconception that a man is in total control over whether he has an erection and that any erection that happens during a session is deliberately caused, there are other common areas of confusion.

Sometimes bodyworkers assume that if a client doesn't say anything or look uncomfortable, that having an erection does not bother him. However, many men say that at such a time, they are embarrassed but decide to keep quiet, hoping the therapist won't notice. You have to remember that even the possibility of having an erection keeps many men from ever seeking a professional massage.

Sometimes practitioners think that if a client is aroused or has made sexual remarks or requests, they (the practitioners) have done something wrong to cause the arousal or that they have somehow given the client a mixed message. Massage therapists can feel a sense of shame at such times, as if they have been encouraging the client in some way. That confusion can make practitioners uncertain about how to respond. Even if there's no hint of inappropriate behavior, when a client is aroused, it can set off questions in the therapist's mind: "Does he think this is a sexual massage? Have I somehow led him to believe that or been seductive in some way?" Especially if you don't know the client well, the situation can be uncomfortable, awkward, and even scary.

Your goal is to protect yourself, your dignity, and your reputation without humiliating a client who means no harm.

First, make an assessment. Is this a natural physiological response, or is the client deliberately arousing himself? What has been your history with this client? If you have no reason to mistrust a client—for instance, you've worked with the client many times before and he's never tried to cross into sexual territory—you might continue working and assume that his response is innocent. However, if this is a new client who has already given you reason to mistrust him or a client who has skirted the edges of decency before, then your choices will be different. Or if you're not sure what the client's intentions are, then you have another course of action.

CLIENTS WHO ARE HAVING A NATURAL,
UNINTENTIONAL RESPONSE

What should you do when you notice that your client has an erection and you're pretty certain that it's just a physiological response? Should you ignore it or say something? And if you say something, what should you say and when should you say it? Is it a good idea to talk with new male clients about the possibility that they could have an erection? All of that depends on the client's behavior, your professional relationship with the client, and your assessment of him. Depending on all that, you have these choices:

Ignore It   Under the theory that what goes up must come down, practitioners often choose to ignore an erection. If the client isn't acting inappropriately, most bodyworkers probably wouldn't interrupt the flow of a massage to talk unless the client says something.

Work on a More Neutral Part of the Body   You can keep doing what you're doing, move to a less intimate part of the body, or ask the client to turn over. Or if you know, for instance, that having work on his abdomen or thighs gets a client stirred up, you can work with that area earlier in the massage when he's less relaxed. You also have the option of avoiding an area the client finds stimulating. However, you don't want to make a practice of limiting the range of your massage simply because of your personal discomfort.

Clear the Air—Say Something   It's not unusual for practitioners, especially women, to be uncomfortable about dealing with a client having an erection. While men and women practitioners seem to feel equally violated by a client who expects sex and is being offensive, men seem to have more locker-room ease with a client who has an unintentional erection. Regardless of your gender, if you think that silence might be adding to your discomfort or the client's, then it's a good idea to clear the air. You can say something such as, "It's really natural for a man to have a physical response to massage."

If you think he's embarrassed or he says he is, you can say, "Oh, that happens. Would you be more comfortable if you turned over?" or "Try focusing on your breathing." Speak in a matter-of-fact way and without disapproval.

Use a Towel   While some suggest that you place a towel over the groin, most think that would only draw attention to the area without communicating a clear message.

CLIENTS WHO ARE QUESTIONABLE OR OVER THE LINE

If you're either not sure of the client's intentions or are pretty sure that his intentions are out of bounds, use the same tactics as for responding to a client who is sexualizing the situation: stop the massage and define your boundaries with a statement such as, "I want to be sure that you know that this is a nonsexual massage. I will end the session if you are looking for something else."

Depending on his response or on your comfort level or your intuition, either state that the massage is over or proceed with caution, letting him know that you will end the massage if he continues being offensive.

EDUCATION BEFORE THE SESSION

Whether to say something before a session begins is a judgment call made on a case-by-case basis. For instance, it might be helpful to talk with a client if he usually gets erections during the massage. Talk with him before he has taken off his clothes or gotten on the table. You could say, "I noticed you had an erection during the last massage, and I wanted to clear the air and say that I know that erections are usually just a physiological response to touch and it's not unusual for clients to have them." If he is a relatively new client, you could add, "Since you're a new client, I want to make it clear that this isn't a sexual massage." A legitimate client shouldn't be offended and might be relieved.

Of course, if a client expresses concern before the massage about having an erection, then you want to educate him that erections can happen without sexual intent and they aren't necessarily a cause for concern. A colleague had a humorous way to clarify the boundaries for a client who asked, "What if I get an erection?" She said, "If you don't pay any attention to it, I won't, either."

Most massage therapists say they don't bring up the possibility of an erection unless the client mentions it. They think that even saying, "You might have an erection" could make a client wonder if you're sexualizing the situation. Of course, that's not always the case. For instance, if a white-haired grandmotherly massage therapist talked to an 18-year-old man about what's normal, he would probably appreciate the reassurance.

SUPPORT AND SUGGESTIONS

If you still find yourself anxious about a client having an erection even though you know it's an innocent response, you could talk with colleagues and mentors for support and advice. Unless you limit your practice to women, you will occasionally encounter erections.

This work is intimate, and nowhere is that more evident than with "the erection dilemma." The potential embarrassments on both sides challenge us to hone our communication and boundary-setting skills. Whether we're dealing with a major creep or a minor "oops," we're called on to use our professional judgment and our common sense. It's all just part of the job.

Protecting Ourselves From Ethics Complaints or Legal Charges

Chapter 5 discusses keeping good framework and boundaries as a way to avoid ethics complaints. This section focuses specifically on ethical issues related to sexual complaints. Although maintaining good boundaries and solid framework are always protection against ethics complaints, some red flags and troublesome situations are unique to sexual issues.

Here are some warnings that may help you make your way through the troublesome situations that can arise:

No One Is Immune

Any practitioner can be complained against by any client. Any practitioner, male or female, gay or straight, can be accused of sexually violating a client. Seductive or careless practitioners are not the only ones accused. Even good-hearted, conscientious practitioners can have clients misread their intentions.

Sexual abuse and violation issues are about power, and they cross all lines of gender and sexual orientation.

Heterosexual women practitioners can be accused by heterosexual women clients, for instance, as the case below shows. Sexual abuse and violation issues are about power, and they cross all lines of gender and sexual orientation. The body holds the unconscious, and the unconscious is often primitive and irrational. That's why we have to provide clear boundaries when we do this work.

> A heterosexual female practitioner was working around a female client's sacrum and was suddenly accused by the client of violating her anally. The practitioner was horrified and immediately removed her hands from the client. She worked the rest of the session to calm the client's concerns, but the client never seemed to regain trust in her and stopped coming for sessions.

In retrospect, the practitioner realized she might have avoided the misunderstanding if she'd taken more care. She was doing deep emotionally oriented work, and she knew this client was fragile and confused about boundaries. There are a number of ways she most likely could have avoided the misunderstanding: (1) by asking the client to leave on her underwear or by working on top of the draping, (2) by getting the informed consent of the client (during the session she could have explained where she wanted to work and the purpose of working in that area and then asked the client's permission), or (3) by postponing the work. (If she thought the client was too deep into an altered state to give informed consent at that point, she could have not worked in that area for that session. Then, at the next session, before the client was on the table, she could explain the possible need to work in that area and asked for the client's consent.)

No one is immune to being misunderstood by a client. However, if you consistently attend to framework and boundaries, you'll be more likely to head off trouble from the start.

Some Are at Greater Risk

Although anyone can be complained against, if you are in a group that is generally perceived as sexually aggressive, whether or not that perception is accurate, you may be more likely to be complained about or sued. Since most complaints are by female clients against male practitioners, men, as a whole, are more at risk. In conservative parts of the country, minority men can be even further at risk, as can homosexual practitioners. All of us who touch people need to be cautious about sexual boundaries, but practitioners in those groups should be extra careful.

Seductive Clients Call for Proper Boundaries

There are instances of seductive clients causing problems for male bodyworkers. (All of the instances I've heard about involve female clients and male practitioners, but the situation could arise between a male client and a female practitioner or between a client and practitioner of the same gender.)

> A male massage school teacher allowed a female client, who had recently been a student in his class, to seduce him. He described that she had "an exquisite sense" of how to connect with him and make him feel special. He said, "She made me feel that making love to her was a heroic and generous act."
>
> But her unbalanced nature soon showed when she began to talk publicly about their sexual relationship as though she had been an unwilling victim. Her stories damaged the teacher's reputation.

Although in this instance, the practitioner did violate his client's sexual boundaries, even practitioners who don't violate boundaries can be falsely accused.

> A male bodyworker described narrowly escaping disaster when a client pleaded with him to have sex with her. She gave him assurances that she wasn't the type to get attached. When he still refused, she retaliated: she went to the police to check the legalities of his license; and she called his landlord and reported he was having wild orgies. None of these actions caused him permanent damage, but he was glad that he had been firm in his refusal.

How do you guard against such emotionally disturbed clients? What are the warning signs? Sometimes you can tell by the feelings these clients bring up in you. One red flag is feeling the need to rescue the client. The bodyworkers in these stories felt they were, as one put it, "nobly responding to the true needs of the client" by becoming intimate. He said, "I thought of my client as an extraordinarily sensitive being who only needed support and recognition to realize her full potential."

When you feel like a noble rescuer, you may be responding to the client's deep need to be saved. This kind of intense transference from a client is highly volatile and can, as the stories show, quickly change to disappointment and rage.

Another warning sign is a feeling of specialness—that either the client or you are special and do not have to stay within normal boundaries. Some mentally unbalanced clients are experts at making practitioners feel special. They know just the right buttons to push.

The intensity of the feelings of specialness goes beyond normal transference. If a client make you feel unusually attractive, competent, or sensitive and is either suggesting that the two of you become lovers or you have started thinking about that possibility, you are in a dangerous situation.

Your countertransference in these cases can feel as if a spell has been cast over you. You can break the spell by getting a good dose of reality from a grounded professional you trust. And you can also remember this: there's never a good reason to have sex with a client or student or even a recent ex-client or ex-student.

Getting a consultation from a trained mental health professional can help you understand the dynamics of the situation. Seductive clients, for instance, do not always want you to be their lover; they're telling you how they habitually deal with power in relationships. They're telling you how they usually get into trouble in their lives or how they get attention. A consultant can help you protect yourself and the client by not playing into the client's unhealthy patterns.

Be Aware of the "Nice Guy" Blind Spot

As well as being aware of clients who may play on our vulnerabilities, we have to be aware of our own blind spots. Many of us don't fully appreciate all the effects of transference; however, the danger is greater for male practitioners who don't have a good enough grasp of this dynamic. If these practitioners don't fully realize the power of women's unconscious attitudes about men and the possible memories of sexual abuse that women may bring to the table, they can be stepping into trouble. Some men may think that because they are "nice guys" or happily married, female clients will somehow automatically feel comfortable with them.

Charles Wiltsie, a massage therapist who conducts ethics classes for male practitioners, says that many men do not understand that the possibility of inappropriate touch and behavior can be quite frightening to many women. Male practitioners, he feels, don't sufficiently understand that for women clients, "The smallest error or slip of a hand can change a relaxing experience into a nightmare."[1]

Similarly, the take-charge behavior that is expected of men in many situations may not serve them well as manual therapists. Here's an example:

> A male massage therapy student was partnered with a female student to learn the techniques for back work. When he began working, he unsnapped her bra without asking her. A teacher noticed both what he'd done and the woman's startled reaction. When the male student was asked to explain his actions, he said, "I thought it would be easier for me to get to her back muscles without the bra in the way."

---

[1] Wiltsie CW III. Uniquely male: Ethics in massage therapy. Massage & Bodywork 1999;April/May:46.

It's understandable for a student to be focused on learning technique, but goal-oriented behavior isn't necessarily helpful in manual therapists. As practitioners, men are safer from misunderstandings if they let the client run the show. Clients need to know they are in charge of what happens, especially when the gender dynamics involve a male practitioner and female client. In this case, for example, the student could have asked permission to unhook the woman's bra, explaining the therapeutic reason for it.

We want to guard against the kind of behavior that could be misunderstood or that could cause us trouble, either the relatively minor trouble of losing a client or the major trouble of a complaint or lawsuit against us.

Protecting the Profession

There are people in every profession who use their roles to take advantage of clients sexually, and ours is no exception. To protect the profession, we need to distinguish between the well-intentioned practitioner who has stumbled into a destructive situation or made a mistake in judgment and the practitioner who habitually seduces clients or violates their sexual boundaries and who is indifferent to the emotional damage he causes.

Predatory Behavior

Predators are practitioners who deliberately and habitually misuse the power of transference to take advantage of their clients. They may be sexually inappropriate during sessions or may make a habit of dating their clients, often secretly dating several at once.

Some clients go along willingly with a predator because they say he makes them feel special and seems interested only in them. For instance, during a session, a practitioner may start by flirting to see if a client is open to further advances and then begin to touch the client with sexual intent. Although the client may not protest at the time, the aftermath often leaves the client feeling violated. She may feel guilty for having flirted with the practitioner and for "leading him on," not realizing that she is not the first and won't be the last client that the practitioner involves in sexual activity. She may be reluctant to make a complaint against him. However, even if the client has appeared to consent at the time, the practitioner has still violated the client's trust and has committed a serious breach of ethics.

Predators can also take advantage of clients without flirting or making the sexual activity appear to be mutual—by deliberately working too close to a client's breasts or genitals, for instance—without the client's informed consent and without therapeutic intention.

Such behavior can be damaging and traumatizing. Over the years, our profession, like the culture in general, has become increasingly sensitive to sexual harassment and misuse of power. In the late 1970s and early 1980s, manual therapists weren't aware, as they are now, that dating a client or flirting with a student was unethical. However, as a profession, we have become increasingly aware of the damage that can be done by crossing these boundaries.

We have also reflected the culture in coming to an understanding that seductiveness isn't about sex and affection; it's about dominance and hostility. Practitioners involved in habitual predatory behavior are often sociopaths, that is, seductive charmers who have no concern about the harm done to others. Habitual predators do great harm to clients and to the reputation of the profession. It's in the interest of the profession to find ways to expose them and shut them down.

No Witch Hunts

I'm not advocating witch hunts. You don't want to be quick to point the finger, jump into lawsuits, or drag people's names through the mud for little or no reason. There's no healing in such actions.

Be very careful about making accusations. Rumors and unsubstantiated gossip can harm the reputation of an innocent person, affecting that person's livelihood. Aside from being unkind and unethical, it can subject you to slander suits from the accused.

When you have reason to question another practitioner's ethics, the decent way to handle it is to approach the practitioner directly in a manner that shows you're looking for information and haven't yet drawn conclusions. The first step is to make a phone call to the person or to write a letter: "I've heard this about you. I thought you needed to know what is being said so that you can respond to it." The practitioner then needs to either deny

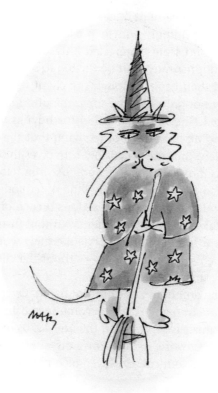

that the rumors are true or explain the circumstances. If this is a practitioner who was just momentarily off balance who gives assurance that such behavior won't happen again, you would probably be right to decide not to take further action.

If the practitioner denies the rumors, but the rumors persist over time, perhaps joined by new ones, then you need to go through the appropriate channels of the relevant professional association or licensing board. In that way, confidentiality is (or should be) guaranteed. Also, if the practitioner doesn't deny the rumors but also does not see the harm in such behavior and can't be persuaded of it, then you would need to let the practitioner know that you'll take further action.

Dealing With Predatory Behavior

Taking action against a predator isn't easy. Predators are a problem across the board—they crop up in all different kinds of manual therapy, regardless of how incompatible their behavior is with the underlying philosophy of their training. Predators give the manual therapies a bad name; they damage the reputation of other practitioners who work near them, especially those who do their brand of work.

I've talked with practitioners all across the country who have tried to stop predators in their bodywork communities and their cities, and the dynamics are very similar—it's usually a difficult process. As happens with other professionals, such suits usually involve female clients and male practitioners. Female clients who have been harassed or mistreated sometimes wrongly feel that they colluded with the predator and are ashamed to take action. Also, women who are taken in by predators are frequently already emotionally fragile and may not make good witnesses—they can be dismissed as "hysterical" or "flaky." The accusers themselves—whether they are the actual victims or those acting on behalf of the victims—can become the target of either hostility or legal action from the accused and from his supporters. This is particularly true if the accuser and the predator are in the same bodywork community. Sides can be taken, and the situation can become divisive.

Even if the accuser isn't under attack himself, taking someone to court or filing a complaint is time consuming and emotionally wrenching. Incidents have to be carefully documented, victims have to be persuaded to participate, and legal advice has to be obtained. The task is difficult. It takes time and energy away from work and personal life, and it requires a good deal of support from colleagues. However, those pursuing such a complaint are performing a service both for the profession and for future would-be victims of that practitioner.

Confusion and Imperfection

Because of the public's misconceptions, manual therapists have to make an extra effort to combat the public misconception that links our work with sexual services. However, we don't need to go too far in the other direction and have unrealistic expectations of ourselves—for instance, to expect ourselves never to have even fleeting sexual thoughts about our clients. We need to be able to be honest with ourselves and each other about our mistakes and humanness.

The sexual issues related to our work can be potentially problematic for manual therapists, as individual practitioners and as a profession. Misunderstandings, inappropriate behavior, and accusations related to sex are the most damaging to both practitioner and to the profession. How do we lower the risk and keep our work environment safe for ourselves and therapeutic for our clients? We should seek outside professional help when we need more clarity about sexual issues that interfere with our work. We need to have more honest discussion among fellow students and colleagues. And we need to soften our attitudes so that we can allow for imperfection and confusion in ourselves and others, while at the same time stopping the behaviors that harm clients.

QUESTIONS FOR REFLECTION

1. If you are a manual therapist or studying to be one, do you have any fears about sexual issues related to this work? What could you do to lessen those fears?

2. Imagine how a female practitioner might feel who is working with a new male client who appears to be having an erection. What would her concerns be? How might she act? Imagine how a man might feel who finds himself having an erection while he is getting a massage from a woman practitioner he does not know well. What would his concerns be? How might he act?

3. Have you ever known of a professional of any kind who was habitually sexually inappropriate or habitually seduced his or her clients? How would you feel about reporting such a person to his or her professional association? What would make you hesitate? What would make you want to go forward?

4. How would it feel to have people assume that because you are a man, a homosexual, or a person of color, you might be more sexually aggressive or less trustworthy than other people? What would you do to combat that image? What could you do to not to take it personally?

5. Do you think you could be easily attracted to a client who acts seductively? Or could you imagine circumstances in your life (being lonely, feeling unsure of yourself because of a recent rejection, and so on) that would make you more vulnerable to such a client? What could you do to keep yourself from acting on such an attraction?

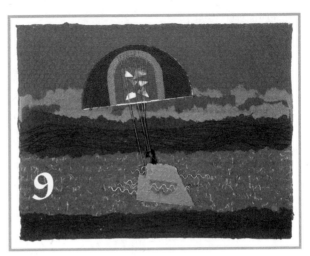

Chapter 9

$\mathcal{F}$INANCIAL BOUNDARIES: GETTING COMFORTABLE WITH MONEY

Many practitioners in our profession are uneasy about the financial side of our work. Most of us don't come to this work with a business background. We spend much of our time in school learning our trade, not learning how to deal with money and fees. However, handling the financial part of our relationship with clients with clarity and grace is an important way that we set safe boundaries for our clients and ourselves.

We may think of the business side of the professional relationship as an unpleasant bit of reality that we tack on to the "true" relationship, the hands-on aspect of our work. But charging a fee (or whatever we ask in return for our work) is actually central to the therapeutic relationship. For the professional relationship to feel safe to clients, they need to know what we expect of them and they need to trust that we will be fair. Also, for the relationship to feel right to us, we need to feel that we are receiving adequate compensation.

This chapter discusses personal issues and attitudes practitioners can have about charging fees that may get in the way of creating effective financial transactions. It is primarily concerned with choices based on individual preference rather than on questions of business ethics.

From Caring One to Cashier: Money Awkwardness

Some of us may feel awkward going from being the one who is compassionate when a client is on the table to being the one who asks for money at the end of the session.

You've just finished a session during which you felt touched by a client's revelation of the pain he feels in his life, and you're feeling compassionate toward him. As he gets ready to pay, he says, "Oh, do you mind if I postdate this check for next week?" Or "Gee, I forgot my checkbook. Mind if I pay you next time?" How do you then say, "I prefer that you pay me at the end of each session" without feeling callous? It might seem easier to say, "Oh, sure . . . that's fine" even if it really isn't fine.

Caring about clients and expecting something in return from them are two different aspects of our relationship with our clients, and we may feel uncomfortable making the transition between the two. Medical doctors and somatic practitioners who do volume business resolve the conflict by having another person, an office manager or receptionist, handle the finances. But most of us are stuck with the dilemma of sliding back and forth between being the caring one and the cashier.

Perhaps we even feel a little guilty about setting fees. A bodyworker said recently, "I'm not in this for the money. This work is like a calling for me." For those with that attitude, there's often an accompanying sentiment that it's somehow crass to care about making money. While there's nothing wrong with wanting to make the world better, there's also nothing wrong with being paid adequately for our work. Part of what being a professional means, after all, is that this is how we pay the rent. Charging appropriate fees tells clients that we respect ourselves and are serious about our work.

For practitioners who are uncomfortable because they feel as if they're charging people for nurturing them or caring about them, a colleague has this advice: "Tell them that clients are paying for their time. The caring is free."

Money as Part of the Healing Process

We have to keep in mind that our fees or compensation are actually an important part of the healing process for clients. Our fees clarify clients' obligations to us and ours to them. Giving a service without making it clear what we expect in return can make both parties uneasy.

It is an intrinsic aspect of clients' healing not only for them to give something in return but also to create a balance by giving something that is valuable to them. Jerome Frank studied many kinds of health care providers—witch doctors, traditional Western medical doctors, and alternative health practitioners. In *Persuasion and Healing*, he discusses his findings that in an effective therapeutic experience, patients or clients must give something valuable in exchange; they must make a sacrifice.[1] In cultures other than our own, the offering might be a nice fat chicken. In ours, it

---

[1]Frank JD, Frank JB. Persuasion and Healing. Baltimore: Johns Hopkins University Press, 1993.

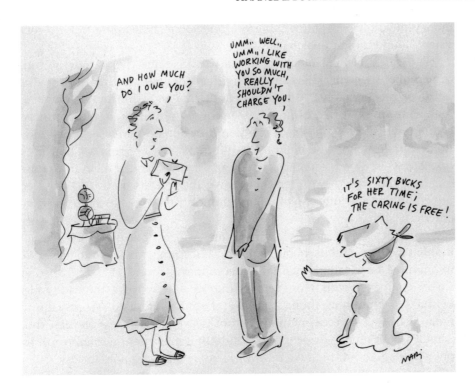

might be volunteering our time so that a new student can practice on us or trading a session with a colleague, but usually what is given is money.

The idea of the healing value of a sacrifice doesn't justify greed or over-charging, but the concept can help us feel more comfortable with collecting appropriate fees. The element of sacrifice may give clients a deeper sense of the treatment's value and help them benefit from it. Many manual thera-pists have discovered that clients who are given a special deal often don't seem to get as much out of the work as those who pay full price.

Although trades can sometimes work out well, money is usually the best way to be compensated. The great thing about money is that it's specific. Sixty dollars isn't the same as $59.75. Money's clean; it's precise; it's simple.

Money's clean; it's precise; it's simple.

The clarity of fees is part of a safe professional environment. They are useful to both practitioner and client. Asking for and receiving money (or whatever the terms of exchange) speaks deeply to both client and practi-tioner about the value of the work. For practitioners, money is a tangible sign of the client's appreciation. For clients, it is a tangible sign of how much they will invest in their own well-being.

Money: An Emotional Issue

As we all know, money can be an emotionally loaded issue. Most people have strong beliefs, opinions, and habits around money. Very few people (especially in the United States) are indifferent to the subject. The fact that both practitioner and client may have strong feelings and attitudes about money makes it both more important and more challenging to keep consistent boundaries in this area.

Regardless of their actual material wealth, some clients may be concerned about whether they are getting their money's worth. They may be sensitive to being slighted on time or effort. They may think our fees are too high. Perhaps not being aware of the expenses of running a small business or the physical and emotional exertion that our work involves, they may think a professional who makes $80 an hour is lavishly paid. Or they may take our fee setting personally, thinking that we don't like them if we raise our fees and we do like them if we give them a discount. (We have to be careful that the latter isn't true and that discounts are based on objective criteria.)

Some of us may have old, unexamined ideas that get in the way of making good decisions about policies concerning money and fees. We might have deep feelings about whether money is "good" or "bad," whether we are competent with it, or even whether we deserve to be financially successful. We might have unrealistic ideas about how hard or how easy it is to make a living. Also, as manual therapists, we work in a profession that usually doesn't make us rich. In a culture that measures personal worth by one's bank account, we have to learn to value our work nonetheless.

Talking to Clients About Money

Because money is an emotional subject for many people, we can quickly offend or even lose a client if we are clumsy in setting limits or unclear about our expectations around fee paying.

Here is a summary of the basic guidelines for setting limits, first discussed in Chapter 6:

- Be clear about expectations in advance.
- Be careful about your tone.
- Speak in terms of your general policy.
- Practice what you will say in various situations.

The importance of these guidelines is worth repeating. First, the clearer you are about what you expect from the beginning, the easier your job will be. Second, when you talk with clients about money policies, your attitude and tone make a world of difference. You want to sound straightforward, businesslike, and confident—neither apologetic nor punitive. Third, when you have to set a limit, if you speak in terms of general policies rather than about a client's specific behavior or circumstance, the client will be less defensive. Instead of saying, "You should have let me know you couldn't come. You have to pay me for the appointment you missed," you can say, perhaps with a sympathetic tone, "As you know, I charge full fee when someone misses an appointment."

The ability to set limits well doesn't come naturally. Just as you use friends and colleagues to practice massage strokes, you can also use them to try out what you will say in different situations. Even though it's a make-believe situation, friends and family can give you valuable feedback about how your words sound and your attitude comes across.

Basic Fee Policies

There are a number of common situations or practices that most practitioners have to deal with around fee setting. As with other aspects of your relationship with clients, it's a good idea to establish fair boundaries and stick with them unless you have a carefully thought-out reason to make an exception.

You also need to be familiar with the appropriate laws in your city or state to be sure you are in compliance with regulations governing various aspects of running a business, such as refund policies, raising fees, marketing, and so forth.

Of course, if you work in a spa or as the employee of a doctor or chiropractor, you probably have to abide by their basic fee policies. It's a good idea to find out whether the employer's policies are fair before you take on a job.

Setting Fees

If you're starting a practice, you can determine the appropriate fee to charge by researching what other practitioners in your community are charging, especially those who offer your kind of bodywork or massage and have your level of experience.

Your rates affect what both clients and colleagues will think about you. If you charge more than the norm, some clients may be put off, while others may think you must be offering something special for the extra charge. If you charge less than the going rate, some clients may be attracted to the bargain but may not value the work as much.

Moreover, if you charge a good deal more or less than what others are charging (say, a difference of $20), you run the risk of alienating your colleagues. Sometimes even a $10 difference in fees can set a practitioner apart. Colleagues may feel you are arrogant if you charge more than they do without having more training or experience. Or they may resent your undercutting them if you charge less than the going rate. On the other hand, if you are a recent graduate, a practitioner new to an area, or even an experienced practitioner whose practice is in a slump, it's acceptable practice to offer a package of sessions at a discounted rate in order to boost business.

The amount you charge also affects how you feel about your work. Make sure that your fees are fair to you and that they take into account all of your expenses—for instance, your office rent; the time and cost of either laundering your own sheets or having them cleaned; and the costs of massage oil, phone service, or even a website. Charge enough so that you won't begin to resent your clients. Also, make sure you don't feel as if you are overcharging. If you're not comfortable with your fees, clients will sense it and feel uncomfortable also.

Raising Fees

How often and by how much practitioners raise their fees can vary. Many raise their fees by $5 or $10 about once a year. Some raise rates when their overhead, such as office rent, becomes higher. To be fair, you need to give adequate notice—a month or two, at least (3 months is standard procedure in Canada)—to let clients get used to the idea of the higher rate and be able to budget accordingly. You can post a notice by your door, so that clients will be sure to see it, or mail a notice to your regular clients. You can also tell them (before they are on the table): "I want to let you know that starting in November, my fee will be $65 instead of $60."

There's a good deal of variation in how you can carry out fee hikes. Some practitioners begin charging the higher fee immediately for new clients but wait a month or two before applying the rate for existing clients. Some never raise rates for existing clients; their clients never pay more than what they paid for their first appointment.

There's no set way to raise fees. Whatever you decide, your policy needs to be one that you can live with, that you feel is fair to you and to your clients, and that you implement consistently. There's no need to feel apologetic about raising your fees. As a colleague said, "We don't need to send clients a sympathy card when we raise our fees."

Special Deals

What about giving discounts or using sliding scales? Many of the practitioners I have talked with find it works best to stick with one fee, with rare exceptions.

As discussed in earlier chapters, making special arrangements for a client in any area of your work generally brings up a red flag. Because money issues are often so emotionally loaded for both client and practitioner, going outside your usual boundaries in fee setting is often a big mistake. It can also be a sign of deeper problems with that client, including allowing a client to manipulate you or feeling guilty about refusing a client.

Giving discounts and charging on a sliding scale are the most common examples of special deals. A colleague reports:

> A prospective client called and said she was under a lot of stress, and she knew it would help her to receive regular massages. She had heard good things about my work but said that massage was "outside her budget" and asked if I would give her a significant discount. Since she was working full time, I told her that I only offered discounts to students and others in special circumstances. When she began pleading with me about how much she needed the work, I almost gave in to her but then realized that I was inappropriately beginning to take on responsibility for her stress level. I told her that I couldn't make an exception for her, and I gave her the names of some practitioners who

> might be willing to give her a discount. Although she was not happy about being refused, I felt that she had not given me a good reason to change my policies—and she had given me good reason to be wary of being manipulated.

You're under no obligation to discount your fees. In many ways, charging everyone the same fee creates the safest, clearest boundaries for both you and your clients. If you do want to consider discounting your fees or making special arrangements from time to time, consider the following points.

KNOW YOUR MOTIVATION

You want to take care that, for one, you're not trying to rescue the client. A "rescue" attitude means you treat the client as if he were in some way inadequate and, therefore, not able to be held to normal business arrangements. Sometimes you may make a special deal because you don't want to say no to a client, you want to be "nice," or you think you need the money, even if it's a lower fee. All of these motivations are different from making an adult-to-adult business arrangement with someone who has a legitimate reason to need a discount, such as an elderly person on a small fixed income. Equally important, when you depart from your normal framework, you encourage clients to do so as well. A colleague reports:

> Even though I don't usually do this, I made a special payment arrangement for a client who said he was down on his luck. He was to receive a ten-session series at the rate of two per month but only pay me for one each month. After we finished the ten, he would continue to pay me a monthly fee until all sessions were paid off. Unfortunately, once we started working, he was an inconsiderate client. For instance, he was often late to sessions, even after I urged him to be on time. Once he missed a session without giving adequate cancellation notice. When we were finished with our work, I had a hard time collecting what he owed me. Lesson learned. I had started out badly with this client by making a special fee arrangement without good cause. I wish I'd noticed then that I had opened myself up to being manipulated.

You can avoid confusion if you have clear guidelines concerning the circumstances under which you will make a special arrangement.

OFFER DISCOUNTS TO GROUPS OF PEOPLE, NOT INDIVIDUALS

Those who do offer discounts often restrict them to certain groups of people, rather than deciding merit on an individual basis. Some school clinics and private practitioners, for example, offer discounts or pro bono work to students, elderly people on a small fixed income, people with life-threatening illnesses, or spiritual or religious teachers. A special fee can work well if it's

A special fee can work well if it's motivated by your heart or your convictions and not by guilt.

motivated by your heart or your convictions and not by guilt. When you make such an exception, you need to keep checking in with yourself to make sure your heart is still in it and your bank balance isn't suffering.

BE WARY OF SLIDING SCALES

Sliding scales are basically discounts, so you need to employ the same caution about using them. Using a sliding scale to determine fees based on a client's statement about his ability to pay automatically creates a dual relationship. In a sense, you become the client's banker, involving yourself in his finances in ways that aren't supposed to be part of your role. You may find yourself concerned about whether the client is spending his money wisely in other areas of his life or whether you should renegotiate his fee if his income rises. The complications created by going outside the boundaries of the therapeutic relationship in this way can interfere with the relationship and with your ability to put your best effort into your work. Imagine these scenarios:

> A client has convinced you that, as a student, she can't afford your full fee. You have agreed to accept $50 per session instead of your usual $80 fee. After you've seen her for a couple of months, she tells you she can't make the next week's regular appointment because she's going on vacation to Hawaii. How do you feel?

> A client who is paying you less than full fee complains after several sessions that she's not getting enough from the work, that she doesn't feel as good as she wants to. Would you be able to handle this complaint with the same objectivity as you would if she were a full-fee client, or might you secretly feel that she's being ungrateful?

ASK YOURSELF SOME POINTED QUESTIONS

Even if you offer to do pro bono or discounted work for what seems like purely altruistic reasons, you want to look at the difficulties that may be hidden in such relationships. Here are some good questions to ask yourself any time you consider reducing fees:

- Do I have a standard policy for fee reduction, and am I veering from that policy?
- Am I reluctant to say no to this client?
- How do I decide how much of a discount to give?
- What are the possibilities that the financial special arrangement will affect the therapeutic relationship?
- Am I expecting special gratitude and appreciation in return for this special fee?

MONITOR THE NUMBER OF DISCOUNTED-FEE ARRANGEMENTS YOU HAVE AT ONE TIME

Determine how many discounted or pro bono (no fee) clients you can realistically afford to see in your practice at one time. You don't want to work all week and end up with little cash to show for it.

It's difficult to make blanket statements about when it's appropriate to give a discount. Some practitioners can handle giving discounts and making special arrangements more easily than others. In deciding what policies you are comfortable with, you have to be honest with yourself about your own limit-setting abilities and your own biases about money. The bottom line is to consider honestly whether the arrangement could be detrimental to you, your client, or the professional relationship.

Common Financial Dilemmas

A number of common situations that arise in the work life of a somatic practitioner can present problems. Although solutions to the problems may vary from practitioner to practitioner, it's best for each practitioner to establish his or her own policy for each of these situations and then stay with that policy.

Missed Appointments

You've booked a new client at 3 p.m. You're not at the movies, you're not taking a nap, you're not attending a class. And most important, you're not able to schedule another client for that time slot. You're all prepared: you've warmed up the room, put clean sheets on the table. Maybe you were counting on the money and you've already mentally spent the fee. And then . . . no client. No phone messages to explain . . . nothing. The missed appointment is that dreadful thud in the professional life of a manual therapist.

The missed appointment is that dreadful thud in the professional life of a manual therapist.

Along with the dreadful thud goes the pesky question of whether to ask the client to pay for the missed session. If the client had a genuine emergency, you wouldn't charge. But what constitutes an authentic emergency? Illness rarely comes on suddenly. Business people usually know that meetings can run long. Sometimes no-show clients can't anticipate problems, but often they can.

In most circumstances, standard practice is to charge a full or partial fee for someone who breaks an appointment without adequate notice or just doesn't show up. (Manual therapists sometimes make exceptions and don't charge the first time a client misses an appointment.) Some practitioners—especially new ones—find it hard to ask a client to pay for a missed appointment. They feel awkward asking payment for "doing nothing." The point is that you could have booked another client in that slot, and even if no other clients wanted that time period, you lost the time it took to prepare and the 20 minutes or so it took to determine that the client wasn't coming.

A missed appointment is time and money lost. Also, if you allow clients to be disrespectful of your time once, chances are they will do it again.

Sometimes practitioners are concerned about making the client angry, so they rationalize that they wouldn't have filled the vacancy anyway. But you have to consider whether you want to work with a client who doesn't respect your time. Also, if you are angry with a client for missing appointments without notice, can you be compassionate when you work with that client?

Sticking to your guns about charging for missed appointments shows that you value your time as a professional. Unfortunately, if the no-show client doesn't call either to explain or to make another appointment and won't return your calls, obviously you can't do anything about it. Such a client probably wouldn't respond to a written bill, either.

To be fair about the adequate-notice policy, you should show clients the same courtesy. Let them know that if you have to cancel an appointment without 24 hours notice, you will give them a free or discounted session. Even with a firm policy that has been communicated to clients, most practitioners have an occasional no-show. Here are some suggestions to make missed appointments less frequent.

SET YOUR POLICY WHEN THE FIRST APPOINTMENT IS MADE

When a client schedules a first appointment, always make sure you let her or him know you will charge for appointments cancelled without 24 hours cancellation notice (or whatever you think is adequate).

PUT IT IN WRITING

During the first appointment, ask clients to sign an agreement accepting the 24-hour cancellation policy (and whatever other policies you have, such as being paid at the time of the session). Even if you are certain you have told clients, they may not remember that you did.

Be sure to include in this agreement the amount of time you will wait—for instance, 20 or 30 minutes—before you decide that the appointment has been missed. Let clients know that it's possible that you might leave the office at that point, so that even if they do finally show up, they may not be able to have even a partial session.

HAVE THE CLIENT CONFIRM

If a client has proved unreliable by missing appointments, ask that client to call you by a certain time the day before the session to confirm the appointment or you will fill that time slot with someone else. (Some bodyworkers ask all clients to confirm the day before.) Or you may prefer to ask permission to call the client with a reminder a day or two in advance.

EXPLORE CREDIT CARD PAYMENTS

If you are able to take credit card payments, you can ensure payment just as other businesses such as hotels do. When a client makes an appointment, take her or his credit card number and let the client know you will charge for a missed session unless the appointment is cancelled by a certain time.

Using the credit card method is particularly useful for those who work a great deal with one-time clients, such as vacationers in resort towns.

Gift Certificates

Some somatic practitioners offer gift certificates as a way to promote business or bring in extra income, especially around the holidays. While they can bring in extra income, gift certificates can also bring some problems.

Many experienced practitioners say that gift certificates are often not worth the trouble. For instance, the giver of the gift may be much more enthusiastic about the benefits of massage than the recipient; the recipient may be reluctant, for whatever reason, to have a massage. As a result, recipients sometimes drag their feet about collecting their massage. Sometimes as much as a year can pass before they make an appointment. Because of this, some practitioners put an expiration date on gift certificates. (In some states, because the service has been paid for, using an expiration date is illegal.) However, most practitioners say they wouldn't turn down such a client regardless of when she or he calls.

Although there are these downsides to gift certificates, they work well for some practitioners. And for some, the process of advertising and selling gift certificates is a good exercise in learning how to promote their businesses.

Refunds

It's often wise to offer a dissatisfied client a full or partial refund even if there has been no negligence or harm on your part. If a client is upset enough to ask for his money back, you're generally better off honoring that request. Aside from wanting to respect the client's wishes, you don't want the bad publicity of an angry ex-client complaining about you to others.

If a client has an unpleasant experience during a session, whether or not you were totally responsible, then you want to make it up to the client. Regardless of whether you had control over the situation that caused a client's discomfort, you bear some of the responsibility. Also, if you want to stay on good terms with the client, refunding all or part of a fee or offering a discount on a future session are good options. Here are two examples:

> A massage therapist charged a client for only half a session when the last 10 minutes of the hour were disrupted by the loud barking of the neighbor's dog.

> A practitioner gave a total refund to a client who had had an allergic reaction to his scented massage oil. Although the client had not told the practitioner that she was sensitive to perfumes, the practitioner was still sorry that the client had had a bad experience and didn't want the client to have a negative feeling about his work.

Certainly, if it *is* your fault that the client feels dissatisfied, you need to offer a full or partial refund:

> A woman had received four sessions from a bodyworker. The bodyworker ended the fifth one 20 minutes earlier than the others, and the client felt the quality of the work was below what she'd come to expect. After leaving the bodyworker's office, she realized she felt shortchanged and called him, explaining what she had noticed. He told her that she was right—that he had been on the verge of catching the flu when he worked with her. He didn't apologize or offer a refund or a discount on another session. Not surprisingly, the client never went back to him and never referred anyone else to him.

This example doesn't mean that whenever you feel you've performed less than your best, you should rush to offer a free session. Those who are very self-critical would be constantly offering free sessions. However, it was the practitioner's responsibility to monitor his own energy level and health and cancel the appointment to avoid giving an inadequate session (and in this case, to avoid the possibility of giving the client the flu).

To guard against an irate client's making a complaint to your professional association or filing a lawsuit, you may need to make it clear in writing that in giving the refund you are not admitting that you have been in the wrong. Also, along with acknowledging receipt of the refund, you may want the client to agree in writing to take no further action and make no further complaints against you. If you have doubts about how best to make a refund without giving the client fuel for further action, you would be wise to get professional legal counsel.

Gratuities and Gifts

Whether to accept gratuities (tips) and whether to accept gifts are two other common money issues.

GRATUITIES

Whether or not to accept gratuities can be a controversial subject for somatic practitioners. Some practitioners question whether it's professional for massage therapists to accept tips because other professionals do not. Most think that practitioners who work for themselves should charge adequate fees and not accept tips. However, for those who work for lower wages in a spa or salon, tips can be a necessary financial supplement.

When tipping is expected, there are ways to make it less confusing and awkward for clients. Customers who receive a massage in a spa or salon often aren't sure whether to tip. The owners should make it clear to them that tips are a normal part of the business by posting a sign on the premises or adding a statement on their list of services: "Gratuities are appreciated." When the practice of tipping is encouraged, it's best if there's an envelope for each employee at the check-in desk (and that the clients know that) so that a practitioner won't necessarily know how much a particular client has given and can concentrate on doing a good job for all clients.

GIFTS

Gifts from clients are a more personal sign of appreciation than tips. Whether to accept gifts needs to be evaluated on a case-by-case basis, taking into consideration the size and value of the gift and what the client's intention seems to be.

Inexpensive gifts given on holidays or special occasions as signs of clients' affection or appreciation are generally fine to accept. You might think twice, however, about accepting frequent gifts, larger gifts, or gifts that you know are an extravagance for the client. Also, if you are uncertain about the intention behind the gift—for instance, if you know a client is interested in dating you and may want to win you over—it would be best to refuse the gift. Clients who give lavish gifts may, at some level, hope for some special treatment in return. Suppose a client who gave you an expensive gift then wanted the work to continue past the end of the hour.

If you want to refuse a gift for whatever reason, you may do so with a smile and a firm, "Thank you for thinking of me. I really can't accept this." Whether to give discounts or refunds, offer gift certificates, or take tips are questions that practitioners have to decide for themselves. Whatever your decision, it always needs to be with an eye toward creating clear and comfortable boundaries for yourself and your clients. The question to ask yourself always has to be, "Will this enhance the therapeutic relationship, or might it hinder it?"

Rewards for Referrals

Is it a good business practice to reward clients or other professionals for referring clients to you in hopes of stimulating more referrals?

Here are two examples:

> Massage therapist Margaret offers a free massage to any client who refers five new clients who make and keep an appointment with her.

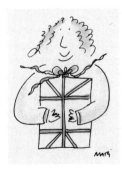

You may not want to accept large gifts from clients.

> Bodyworker Bruce has an arrangement with a chiropractor (for whom Bruce does not work) to give the chiropractor $10 for each new client the chiropractor refers.

These practices are known as "kickbacks" and are both unprofessional and unethical. Prospective clients need to be able to assume that the person recommending you is doing so because he appreciates your competence and skill, not because he is getting a fee or a service in return. Even though the referrer may appreciate your abilities, the reward can influence his judgment.

As a professional, you should expect that clients and other professionals will find your work valuable and want to tell others about it. Although you want to be courteous and thank them for any referrals, a professional should not be in the position of seeming overly grateful for a referral; actually, it is the referrer who should feel grateful for having a skilled and trustworthy practitioner to whom to refer friends and colleagues.

Becoming More Comfortable With Money

Sometimes we graduate from our manual therapy training expecting that we should be able to easily make a good living with our work. However, it may take a while for this expectation to become a reality, and we can feel isolated in grappling with the situation. It's rare for people to share the details of their financial struggles with others, so we may not realize that other practitioners are often having the same problems.

It's not unusual for practitioners to occasionally make mistakes in dealing with clients about money. At some point in their careers, most practitioners have backed down from charging a client for an appointment cancelled at the last minute, for example, or given a special discount that backfired, or undercharged or overcharged a client.

There are ways that we can become more secure with financial dealing. We can first examine our own attitudes about money. Having **mentors** who are comfortable in their relationship to money can be a major help with business issues. Because just about everyone has some issues about money and business, peer group discussions can also be helpful. In a group, one person will have clarity about an issue that another struggles with. Personal supervision can also aid us in getting to the deeper issues that we have about money. (Peer groups and supervision are discussed more fully in Chapter 11.)

Some manual therapists are starting to use coaches—individuals specifically trained to help practitioners create business goals that suit their values. A coach can help us figure out the steps to reach those goals and then, like a personal exercise trainer, hold us accountable for making progress.

Some workshops specialize in improving attitudes about money. To find a good workshop or coach, seek out recommendations from satisfied customers. For practical advice and legal information, it's useful to attend a

Mentor:
A trusted colleague who provides guidance and education. Mentors are usually helpful in advising on both the details of establishing oneself as a professional and the broader general aspects of taking on a professional role or of taking on the role of a particular kind of bodywork or massage practitioner.

workshop, such as one at a local community college, about how to run a small business.

The ability to set good money boundaries is a crucial part of our work. Clients need the comfort and safety of a clear financial relationship, and so do we. Keeping clean and clear about money is, like most boundary issues, a skill and an art that we will practice and improve throughout our careers.

QUESTIONS FOR REFLECTION

1. Fill in the blank with the first words or phrases that come to mind: In my life, money is _____. (You may have several answers.)

2. Think about how or where you may have gotten the feelings or thoughts about money that you wrote in question #1. Did they come from your family? From the culture? Do those answers reflect the attitude you want to have about money? If not, what attitude would you like to have? Fill in the blank to reflect that attitude: I want money to be _____.

3. Do you think it's true that clients will value a service according to what they pay for it? For instance, will they value a service they pay for more than a free one? Will they value a more expensive service over a less expensive one? For instance, if a massage costs $10 rather than $60, will that make a difference in how the client perceives the service? Why or why not?

4. Draw up a list of money policies that you would be comfortable with as a practitioner. If you are already in practice, are there any changes you would make to your current policies?

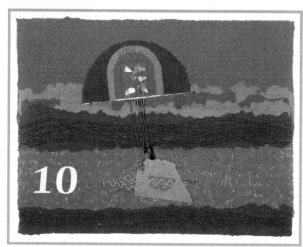

Chapter 10

DUAL RELATIONSHIPS AND BOUNDARIES: WEARING MANY HATS

Dual relationships:
Having a relationship with a client other than the contractual therapeutic one, such as having a client who is also a friend, family member, or business associate.

Dual relationships—having more than one kind of relationship with a client, such as being friends with a client or trading sessions with a colleague—are practically a tradition in our profession. We almost feel as if we have a right to them. Some of us become indignant at the thought of limiting or eliminating dual relationships: "What! I can't have coffee with a client?" "My buddy Bill has been coming to me for years, and it's just fine." "Where would I get clients if not from people I know?" However, many experienced therapists have discovered that such relationships can be more troublesome than they at first appear.

Dual Relationships: Complicated Dynamics

Dual relationships can seem so easy—it can feel natural to become friends with a likable client. It can seem logical to work with friends and family— who better to share our gifts with than people we already love? However, the confusion of changing roles and the power of transference and counter- transference can add complications.

When we try to become friends with Client Carrie, who knows us as Selfless Susie, the always-caring massage therapist who focuses solely on Carrie's needs, it may be hard for her to get used to Civilian Susie, who is sometimes grumpy, insensitive, or needy herself. Or when Big Sister Samantha, who knew us when we were throwing baby food on the floor, becomes Client Samantha, she may have trouble taking us seriously. With dual relationships, each person must shift back and forth between an existing role and a new one, and the transition is not always smooth. More often than not, it is messy and can lead to misunderstandings and stress in our practices.

Here's an example:

> A massage therapist decided to barter with an old friend—she would give him massages, and he would paint her living room. He wasn't a professional painter, but she thought he could do a good job, and he was willing to do the exchange.
>
> As the work progressed, she became unhappy with both her own behavior and the painter's. They both began treating sessions like social visits. She found herself talking about their mutual friends or her own concerns during sessions. His behavior was equally casual—he usually showed up late for his massage appointments and then made business calls on his cell phone before getting ready for the session. Because he was a friend, she had a hard time asserting herself about his loose time boundaries.
>
> To make matters worse, she was unhappy with the quality of his painting work. When he'd finished the living room, she told him that she felt his work was inadequate. He was surprised and offended and only reluctantly repainted part of it. She ended up feeling dissatisfied, he felt offended, and their friendship suffered.

We can't know all the reasons for this unhappy outcome, but it was no doubt complicated by the effects of transference. The painter said later that he had become accustomed to seeing his friend as the nurturer. He had come to expect her to take care of him, forgetting that he had an adult responsibility for his side of the bargain. He then felt hurt when she criticized his work. When we are switching roles, the effects of transference and countertransference can create confusing situations.

In this story, we also see examples of two problems that are discussed later—how easy it is for both parties to be casual about framework when we are working with friends and the difficulty of **bartering** services or doing **trades**, especially with someone who is not trading his or her own professional services.

Many experienced practitioners stay clear of dual relationships because of the built-in problems. Whether we're trying to turn a client into a friend, doing a trade, or any of the other possibilities, both sides can end up feeling shortchanged.

Bartering: Exchanging a manual therapy session for goods or services other than another manual therapy session.

Trade: Exchanging a manual therapy session for a manual therapy session with a colleague.

Common Problems With Dual Relationships

Here are the most prevalent kinds of dual relationships and how they can be problematic.

Becoming Friends With Clients

It's not unusual for clients to want to become friends with us. Clients feel the heart connection in our work and want that connection to extend outside sessions. We may feel the client's affection toward us and mistakenly think that affection should be carried into our daily lives rather than remain as part of the professional relationship, where it belongs. Or perhaps we find ourselves really liking a client and wanting to build that into a friendship. Despite those feelings, it's often a mistake to try to change the therapeutic relationship into a social one.

The effects of transference can make it hard to ever have an equal relationship. Because clients often give more weight to what we say and do, it may be unrealistic to expect them to adjust to the normal give and take of a friendship. On some level, clients usually have difficulty seeing us as real people with flaws and our own concerns. Even outside the office, they may expect us to be always focused on their needs, as we are during a session. There is also a chance that they would always see us as better or wiser than they are and that we would exploit that in some way.

Socializing with clients should occur rarely, if at all. Feldenkrais instructor Paul Rubin says, "If you're finding a number of friends through your practice, something is out of balance. Whose needs are being met?"

There is also the possibility that we would disappoint the client by showing our humanness. A colleague reports:

> A client I had seen for several months asked me to have lunch with her, and we began to socialize. Prior to that, she had been an enthusiastic client—she saw massage as part of a new, healthier way of life, and she saw me as part of this new and exciting direction. Unfortunately, as she got to know me, she found out that I wasn't as perfect in my life style as she had imagined—for instance, occasionally I eat junk food. She became disillusioned and discouraged about me and stopped making massage appointments.

Befriending some of our clients can also interfere with our relationships with other clients. They may hear about these friendships and become jealous or uncomfortable about the limits of our boundaries.

Here are some guidelines for dealing with the temptation of becoming friends with clients.

ASK YOURSELF IF THE CHANGE IN ROLES WOULD BENEFIT THE CLIENT

Be sure you're not using the client. When you're tempted to become friends with a client, ask yourself if changing the boundaries of the therapeutic relationship truly helps the client or primarily fulfills your needs.

Here is a colleague's experience:

> I never socialize with my clients or even ex-clients, so I was surprised to find myself thinking about asking my ex-client Mary to attend a concert with me. I realized that I was drawn to this unusual boundary bending because I was lonely. A good friend had recently moved away, and I had a gap in my social life. I felt tempted to fill it with an ex-client I really liked. Once I realized what the problem was, I began thinking of other ways to find new friends.

EVALUATE WHETHER THIS CLIENT COULD EVER SEE YOU AS AN EQUAL

Honestly ask yourself whether the client could ever be a friend with you or whether that client has you on a pedestal. A colleague reports:

> I was thinking of accepting the invitation of a client to attend a movie together. I liked this client and sensed that she wanted to be friends, but I was concerned that if she saw me in my day-to-day life, I might do something that would interfere with the professional relationship, such as saying something that would hurt her feelings When I expressed my doubts to her, she said, "Oh, I know it'll be okay to be friends. I know you would never do anything that would be harmful to me." Her saying that helped me see how idealized I was in her mind. I knew we could never really be friends. I had to tell her that I thought it would be best to stick with my policy of not socializing with clients.

SOCIALIZE WITH THE CLIENT, BUT KEEP YOUR PROFESSIONAL ROLE

Sometimes it's not a problem to socialize with clients or ex-clients if practitioners remain aware of their roles and responsibilities.

Vivien Schapera, the director of Alexander Technique of Cincinnati, says that although she does not initiate social invitations, she does sometimes accept one from a client. She has wise advice about socializing with clients and former clients:

> We can be social, but we can't show what I call our "lower selves." We can't show our pettiness, neediness, jealousies, etc. We tend to work from our higher selves, so clients tend to think we are better than we really are. We may thrive on this adulation. However, once we become friends with our clients, we may find ourselves resorting to our lower selves in the same way we do in the comfort of our own homes and with our closest friends.

> If we get into a difficult situation with a friend who is also a client, if they push our buttons, we have to pull ourselves out of being 3 years old, regardless of how justified we might feel. We must remember that we are the practitioner, always. It never goes away. No matter how hard it is, we have to be "big," we have to be the role model, we have to be generous, we have to give the benefit of the doubt, etc.
>
> It's a delicate and fragile thing to have multiple roles. So if we take someone on as both a client and a friend, we are never justified in letting them down.

LEARN HOW TO TURN DOWN INVITATIONS

Practitioners can feel awkward or unkind when they have to refuse a client's invitation. It's a good idea to assure them that it's part of your professional policy, not a personal rejection. You can say, " Thank you so much for thinking of me; however, I have a policy of never socializing with clients. The relationship we have is special and important for the work that we do together. It would change if we tried to take it outside these walls. I hope that you understand."

Working With Friends and Relatives

There are several reasons why it's not a good idea to work with friends and relatives. Professionals need to work with an objective, nonjudgmental attitude and not have their own agendas for a client. Clients need to be able to focus on themselves and not be aware of our needs. These goals are impossible when we work with people who are involved in our lives in other ways.

Here's an example of having a personal agenda:

> Your friend Bill is very uptight about his job these days. Aside from being concerned about him, you want him to lighten up because he's not fun to be around. When he comes in for a massage, you are highly motivated to get him to relax. Rather than gently coaxing him to let go at his own pace, as you would any other client, you try to force his muscles to soften. Your haste says, "Hurry up and relax, Bill!" However, it's hard for him to let go because he senses your impatience. It's a frustrating experience for both of you.

We can also take friends for granted and not give them the same courtesies we give other clients:

> Your friend Heather comes to you as a paying client because she's stressed out. You've got some errands to do before the session, and since it's *just* Heather, you know you can start late. Also, you haven't seen her for a while, so you use the session time to catch her up on your news. Is that fair to Heather?

Working with people they know can be hard on practitioners, too. Friends and family don't always appreciate the amount of time, energy, and money we've put into learning a skill that's now intended to support us. They may think that what they're receiving is just a friendly back rub. Also, friends often don't give us the respect we deserve or take the work as seriously as they would with someone they don't know. They may show up late, not call to cancel, or, especially if we work at home, want to hang around after their sessions.

Occasionally, we can make exceptions, but not often. We can sometimes see a friend or family member on a one-time or occasional basis and not have problems, but we have to give serious consideration to whether we want to work with a friend regularly.

Mixing Social Occasions With Work

Just as we don't want sessions to be about socializing, social gatherings aren't an appropriate place to display our professional talents. Even students who don't charge for their work shouldn't comply with requests to rub a sore shoulder outside of an office or workspace. (An exception can be made for students who get together after school to socialize. The social occasions discussed here are those with prospective clients.) It sets a bad precedent to work during our off-hours.

It can be difficult to turn down friends who want free samples, but we can just smile and say, "I'm off duty," or "Do you want to set up a time to come see me in my office?" Friends and family need to know that it's unfair to ask us to be available all the time. Also, we can tell them that we can do a better job in a professional setting when our attention can be focused

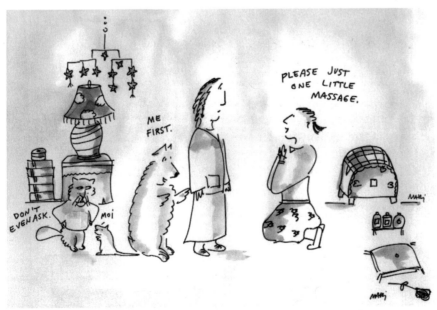

It can be difficult to say no to friends who want "free samples."

solely on them—which is true. The same applies for consulting at a party about someone's bad back. It's tempting to want to show off or sell our work in a social gathering, but it's not an appropriate place for a professional consultation. We can simply give out our business card and ask the person to call during business hours. We can say, "I'd really like to discuss it with you, but I can't really do you justice in an atmosphere like this. How about calling me on Monday, and I'll be glad to talk with you more."

The Complications of Trades and Bartering

Trades and bartering used to be seen as a charming hippie sort of thing, a way to bypass the supposed crassness of money, a way to live more simply. Some people still feel that way about bartering and trading services and goods. However, trading and bartering have the potential for being real pains in the neck and sources of misunderstanding, especially if they are on-going rather than one-time practices. Many of the practitioners I interviewed have discontinued doing trades or barters.

Trading and bartering are problematic because, along with having the potential confusion of changing roles, they lack the clarity and simplicity of a money exchange. We have to work harder to be sure that each side is happy with what is received and each feels the exchange to be balanced. Here's an example:

> Mary agrees to an ongoing trade of massage with her colleague Donna, but as the exchange progresses, Mary feels less and less satisfied. Although Mary treats Donna as she would a regular client, Donna doesn't do the same. She's never on time, she interrupts the massage to take phone calls, and she seems halfhearted in her efforts.

In general, trading for bodywork or massage is more likely to be a problem than bartering, when we exchange our work for a tangible object or a service other than bodywork. The intimacy of our work and the possibilities of transference and countertransference can make trading sessions more difficult. When we trade bodywork, each person finds out about the other's physical and sometimes personal problems. That can interfere with how the person who is the client experiences the massage. For instance, if you know that your practitioner has a persistent wrist problem, would you ask her to go deeper? If you know that she's upset over her divorce, would you complain if she were late for your massage?

Here are some ways to minimize the confusion when doing trades and bartering.

DO ONLY ONE-TIME TRADES

Trades have a better chance of working if they are one-time-only practices and not ongoing. For instance, many practitioners who are new in a community trade sessions as a way to introduce their work to other practitioners.

BE CLEAR ABOUT THE DETAILS OF THE TRADE FROM THE BEGINNING

The challenge with trades is to be very clear what the exchange is. It's best to write it down for both parties to see. Some practitioners say they don't like doing trades because they often end up trading one of their $70 sessions for someone else's $50 session. You can trade two sessions for one or one and a half sessions for one, but the point is to enter into the exchange knowing exactly what the trade is and that both parties are satisfied with it.

BE CAREFUL IF YOU BARTER FOR A SERVICE RATHER THAN FOR SOMETHING TANGIBLE

Some forms of barter are off-limits. For example, bartering for psychotherapy isn't generally considered legitimate in the professional psychotherapy community. But what about bartering for other services? One of the difficulties is in being precise. Suppose you're bartering a session for 2 hours of house cleaning. The client's idea of how a house should look after 2 hours of cleaning can be different from yours. If it's not as tidy as you want, then it's awkward to switch from the nonjudgmental practitioner role to that of the complaining customer. It's also less than desirable for a client to have such an intimate glimpse of your private life and personal habits. A colleague says, "I don't want clients to see what's inside my car—all the clutter and junk food wrappers—much less what's inside my house."

However, it can work to barter for other services that have a set fee and are not highly personal, such as bartering for yoga classes.

BE CLEAR ABOUT VALUE WHEN BARTERING FOR GOODS

The happiest exchanges can be for various goods, particularly artwork. It's important that the value of the item be clear and agreed upon by both parties beforehand. Also, if you're bartering for something you haven't seen, you may want to negotiate what will happen if you don't like the finished product.

SPELL OUT HOW TO TERMINATE THE AGREEMENT

Be clear ahead of time about how to work things out if one of the parties decides to quit before the exchange is even. Suppose a practitioner is bartering Healing Touch for tap dance lessons. She's given $200 worth of Healing Touch sessions and has only received $100 worth of dance lessons. At that point, she decides she doesn't want to be the next Bojangles and doesn't want any more lessons.

Because they hadn't already resolved how to handle this possibility, they now have some potentially sticky questions to resolve. Since she is the one who changed her mind, does the dance teacher owe her anything? And if he does owe her the $100 balance, does he have to pay it all immediately? The details can vary, but it's best to work them out ahead of time. Putting them in writing makes clear that you both understand the terms.

IF POSSIBLE, TRADE OR BARTER WITH PROFESSIONALS

It's easiest to trade with someone who is a professional at whatever the service or work is. Professionals usually have a clear idea of their prices and know how to work with clients.

BE WILLING TO SAY NO

Don't agree to a trade or barter just to please or to take care of someone else, and don't barter for something unneeded or unwanted.

Don't agree to a trade or barter just to please or to take care of someone else, and don't barter for something unneeded or unwanted. These situations are uneven from the start and can breed resentment. You should also be careful about how many such exchanges you take on at once so that you are not working all week and ending up with no cash. Remember that trades and barters can take more energy than regular clients because of the time spent negotiating terms as well as the likelihood of misunderstandings.

Despite all the possible problems, trades sometimes work out well. Some practitioners have established workable trades with colleagues, often those who were fellow students, in which the trade feels mutually beneficial and the two also give each other valuable feedback.

Business Relationships

The ethics of selling products to clients or involving them in business deals is covered in more detail in Chapter 5 on Ethics. To review, there are two main problems:

1. Because of transference, the client may not be as free as a nonclient to refuse to buy whatever the practitioner is selling. Even just a suggestion from a respected or beloved practitioner can feel like an offer the client can't refuse.

2. If something goes wrong—the lotion is messy, the stocks drop, the pillow doesn't seem to help the neck pain—the client may not feel as free as a nonclient to complain or ask for a refund. And you could lose a client if a business deal or product doesn't pan out.

Involving clients in other business transactions can cause resentment, lower the client's respect for the practitioner, and interfere with the therapeutic relationship.

Just as we don't want to engage clients in business, we want to be careful about taking on business associates as clients. Here's the kind of confusion that can happen:

> A massage therapist who is a part-time operating room nurse gave a massage to one of her nursing colleagues. During the massage, when the colleague talked about problems she was having at home and cried, the therapist was appropriately sympathetic and understanding. After that, the colleague started slacking off at work. She excused herself for not doing her part by saying to the nurse/massage therapist, "I know you understand what a hard time I'm having these days."

Practitioners also report having problems when they work with someone who is their boss or has authority over them in another setting. For instance, sometimes bosses want to continue acting as if they are in charge when they become clients. They can be demanding clients, expecting to be given extra time or special concessions. Setting limits with the boss or even contemplating having to set limits can be uncomfortable.

Also, sometimes practitioners rightfully do not wish to know the people for whom they work that intimately or are afraid the boss might make an inappropriate comment or sexualize the situation.

Minimizing Problems

It's often hard to avoid dual relationships. Sometimes we have good reason to take on a friend as a client, do a trade, barter, or even socialize with an ex-client. For example, we may be the only one in town who practices a particular kind of bodywork, and a friend would greatly benefit from that method. We may be the only massage therapist that a shy friend would be comfortable seeing. We may be part of a small community in which it's hard to avoid social contact with our clients.

When are dual relationships likely to lead to trouble, and when might they work? How can we manage dual relationships with the least stress to clients and to ourselves?

Dual Relationships to Avoid

There are a number of circumstances in which a dual relationship would be likely to lead to problems or be harmful to the client.

WORKING WITH FRIENDS OR RELATIVES WHO ARE
IN PHYSICAL OR EMOTIONAL CRISIS

The likelihood of intense transference or dependency when a friend or relative is in crisis makes it difficult to work well with that person. Also, we

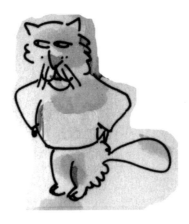

generally have too much investment in such people to have the objectivity to be helpful. A colleague reports:

> My friend had a chronic back problem that flared up right before a vacation. I really wanted to help her. In spite of my best efforts, after an hour she was still in a good deal of pain. Had she been a regular client, I would have been concerned, but I probably would have been able to be more objective. I would have stopped at the end of an hour, knowing that I had done my best and that there may be other factors involved, such as emotional issues. But since it was my friend, I kept trying, which only seemed to make things worse. The fact that I couldn't help her was hard on our friendship, and it took a while for us to be able to talk honestly about what happened.

DOING EMOTIONALLY ORIENTED OR PSYCHOLOGICALLY ORIENTED BODYWORK

Practitioners of emotionally or psychologically oriented bodywork should avoid dual relationships. These practitioners are always working with deep transference issues and cannot risk the complications that would arise from dual relationships.

As with other dual relationships, people who do emotionally oriented work cannot become friends with clients and can rarely become friends with ex-clients. Rob Bauer, a Rubenfeld synergist, says, "People get into emotional issues with Rubenfeld, and transference can happen very quickly, in just one session. For that reason, I don't work with friends or make friends of clients."

HAVING SEXUAL RELATIONSHIPS WITH CLIENTS

As discussed in Chapter 7, maintaining ethical boundaries means that sexual relationships with clients are forbidden and those with ex-clients are limited.

BRINGING CLIENTS INTO OUTSIDE BUSINESS DEALS

As discussed in Chapter 5, involving clients or ex-clients in another business relationship can be unethical.

Tips for Working With Dual Relationships

Here are suggestions for making dual relationships less of a problem.

DISCUSS YOUR MISGIVINGS WITH THE PROSPECTIVE CLIENT

If friends or family members want to work with you, talk with them about the problems with changing roles. Let them know they would probably benefit more from going to a practitioner they don't know. If you both still want to proceed, check in with them regularly to make sure no problems are arising.

KEEP YOUR USUAL BOUNDARIES AND FRAMEWORK STANDARDS

Because you're already bending boundaries by working with someone you know in another way, you need to be more aware of all other boundaries and framework, not less. You may be tempted to think, "Oh, it's just old Bob. I can still be eating my sandwich when he arrives." That would give Bob a message that the setting is not quite professional or safe for him. Aside from interfering with his ability to relax, it's bad advertising for you. Every client is a potential source of referrals; if someone asks Bob how he liked his massage, you want him to endorse you with enthusiasm rather than think, "I hope she acts more like a professional when she's with other clients."

KEEP CONFIDENTIALITY AND SESSION BOUNDARIES

Assure clients with whom you have another relationship that what they say and do inside a session will be held in confidence. Let them know that it's best for the two of you to keep work-related questions and comments inside the office space.

SEPARATE SOCIAL TIME AND PROFESSIONAL TIME

Advise clients that they will get more out of their sessions if you don't mix session time with either socializing or doing business—if you don't chitchat during sessions, talk about business, or go to lunch together right before or after sessions. You might want to stop seeing a friend socially while he or she is a client or, at the very least, not take the friendship to another level. If someone is, for instance, a friend that you see socially every few months, you don't want to start having lunch once a week during your work together.

Special Considerations for Students

It's particularly common for students to work with friends and relatives while they are learning their trade. Although this is not usually a good idea for a professional practice, this can be a useful way for students to acquire experience, become accustomed to doing a certain number of sessions a week, and practice their "bedside manner."

Even in a practice situation, the problems of dual relationships arise. Dianne Polseno, ethics columnist for the *Massage Therapy Journal*, quotes a massage student: "No one's talking about the real issues. I certainly know not to date or sleep with a client. What I don't know is how to handle the 'little things' that crop up when I massage relatives and friends. For me, this is one of the most stressful aspects of my work."[1]

The same "little things" that come up for students also come up for more experienced professionals when they have dual relationships—keeping a friend's massage from becoming a social occasion, dealing with friends who expect a free foot massage, and so forth. However, these situations are more common and troublesome for students who are starting their practices and may feel insecure about claiming a professional role and setting appropriate boundaries.

---

[1]Polseno D. Ethically speaking: Multidimensional relationships. Massage Therapy Journal 1999;Winter;38:113.

Here are some suggestions to help students start out on the right foot.

SET BOUNDARIES FROM THE BEGINNING

When you begin to do practice sessions with friends and family, let them know what to expect from the beginning. You can say, for instance, "I appreciate your being a guinea pig now as I'm learning my trade, and the session will be free. When I've graduated, I'll charge all my clients $60" (or whatever amount you plan to charge).

It's up to you to let friends and family know the boundaries. They may not realize that they're taking advantage of you.

It's easier to set limits at the time the initial appointment is arranged, not after frustration has built because a friend has stayed for 2 hours after her massage. "I'll have an hour available from 2 to 3 o'clock, and then I'll have to take care of some other business." It's up to you to let friends and family know the boundaries. They may not realize that they're taking advantage of you.

TREAT FREE SESSIONS AS IF THEY WERE
"REAL" SESSIONS—PRACTICE BOUNDARIES

A good way to develop professionalism and help the boundaries stay clear is to treat each session as if the client were paying. Let friends and family members know that they will be treated as regular clients and explain what that means: you want to start and end on time; you'll use appropriate draping; and they may talk if they want, but you won't respond in the way that you would in a social situation. You can explain that this framework is helpful to you as a student and will also help them get the most out of their sessions. An added bonus is that friends and family members will have the experience of seeing how professional you've become and will be more inspired to recommend you to someone else.

Be Wary of Dual Relationships

Sometimes we're lucky and squeak by without problems with a dual relationship. Usually, though, these relationships lead to anything from minor annoyances (putting extra energy into sorting out misunderstandings) to major problems (being in hot water for unethical behavior). Clients who are entangled in dual relationships with us often don't benefit from our work as much as other clients do. There just isn't the same amount of attention and therapeutic focus.

Decisions about whether to take on a person as a client need to be based on solid professional judgment, not ease and convenience. However despite the drawbacks, dual relationships will probably always be with us. It helps if we realize the problems intrinsic to their nature and take extra precautions to make the professional relationship safe for both parties.

QUESTIONS FOR REFLECTION

1. Outside of massage or bodywork, have you ever been part of a dual relationship with a friend or family member? How did it work out? If it worked out well, what do you think made it successful? If not, what got in the way?

2. Have you ever been part of a trade? Were you satisfied with what you received from it? If not, what would have made it better?

3. Have you ever been in a situation with a professional or a businessperson in which there was a dual relationship? Were there any problems related to the dual relationship? If not, what do you think helped? If there were problems, what would have helped lessen or eliminate them?

4. At a social occasion, have you ever gotten involved in essentially giving a free consultation or sample of your work to a potential client? How did that work out? If it worked out well, what made the difference? If not, what would you do differently to avoid problems next time?

5. Have you ever gone from being a client to being a friend of a professional of any kind? Were there any issues to work out—for instance, were you disappointed when you found out more about the professional? If it has worked out well to be a friend, do you think that it would always work out well to become a friend of the professionals in your life? Why or why not? If it didn't work out well, what made the difference?

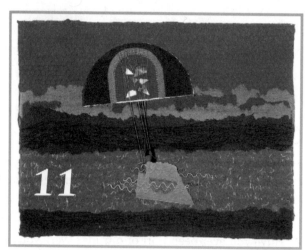

Chapter 11

*H*ELP WITH BOUNDARIES: SUPPORT, CONSULTATION, AND SUPERVISION

Few of us have training in professional relationship skills. True, our common sense and natural instincts are often enough to get us by, but to become solid professionals, we often need outside help and support.

Support can help keep our spark and enthusiasm for our work alive, and that can make a difference in how well we keep boundaries. Learning how to practice good boundaries isn't merely a question of memorizing rules; we can know what we're supposed to do and still make mistakes. How well we maintain boundaries can depend on our overall emotional health and even how we're feeling on any particular day. Discouragement, loneliness, and boredom take their toll on boundary skills. Perhaps the reason for the most common boundary problem—practitioners using clients as a captive audience—comes from the fact that many practitioners feel isolated and want someone to talk with.

Nobody tells us this in school, but it can be lonely out there.

Nobody tells us this in school, but it can be lonely out there.We tend to work in isolation—in our homes, in a private office—and we're alone with clients who may be needy or hurting and looking to us for relief.

Most somatic practitioners find that this work isn't as simple as just giving a rubdown. We work every day with issues of intimacy, dependency, and pain. We all have unresolved beliefs and attitudes that can get in our way. For instance, some of us were raised to believe that we shouldn't complain about aches and pains, that suffering in silence shows strength. How will we feel about clients who come in with a long list of complaints—as is their right? Some of us were brought up to feel that taking care of ourselves and saying no to others is selfish. How well will we then draw the line when a client with a sore back wants an appointment on our day off?

How well we handle the relationship aspect of our work and how much safety we provide for ourselves and our clients can make or break our practices. We need to build into our work lives an abundance of ways to get support, feedback, and new perspective.

There are several options for help: **consultation**; clinical **supervision**, both in groups and individually; peer support groups; peer supervision groups; and mentoring. Since most of these are new ideas for the profession, this chapter explores them in detail.

> **Consultation:**
> A meeting with a professional trained in psychological dynamics to get advice and insight about a particular client or issue.
>
> **Supervision:**
> An ongoing arrangement made with a professional trained in psychological dynamics for help with the relationship aspects of a practitioner's work.

Basics of Consultation, Supervision, and Groups

Many practitioners are learning how to untangle client relationships by consulting with another professional. This might be a one-time consultation about a perplexing situation or ongoing supervision for support and insight.

The consultant or supervisor should be someone who is both experienced in psychological dynamics and appreciative of the issues involved in bodywork and massage therapy. That would be either a bodyworker or massage therapist who also has training or credentials in relationship dynamics or a mental health practitioner who respects the special problems associated with bodywork and massage therapy. A consultant or supervisor doesn't need to be trained in bodywork or massage techniques, since technique won't be discussed. (See "Choosing a Consultant or Supervisor" later in this chapter.)

Consultation

In a consultation, you and your consultant meet outside the session to discuss a particular client or situation. Although the professional might be a psychotherapist or counselor, this kind of consultation isn't the same as psychotherapy. The purpose is to deal with work-related issues. Although you might discover your countertransference issues, personal subjects won't be probed to the same depth as they would be in psychotherapy. Here are some examples of how a consultant could help:

> Massage therapist Mary dreads the days when she sees her client Fred, who constantly complains about his life. Try as she might to be patient, Mary always ends up feeling irritated by his negative outlook.

In this case, a consultant might, for instance, help Mary realize that Fred reminds her of her father, who disappointed her with his sour outlook on life. Simply having an awareness of how she might be transferring feelings about her father to her client could help Mary work with the client more objectively and compassionately. (If this were psychotherapy, Mary would probably be urged to explore her history and feelings about her father in greater depth.) Also, having that insight would probably help Mary to respond more positively when other clients turn out to be complainers.

> Bodyworker Bob has a client who sometimes cries about her failing marriage during her sessions. Lately, she has seemed more depressed, crying frequently and saying she feels hopeless. Bob wants the client to feel free to express her emotions with him, but he has never been entirely comfortable with her crying, and he now feels overwhelmed by her despair. He thinks she should see a counselor but doesn't know how to suggest that without hurting her feelings or making her feel rejected.

There are several issues that Bob could discuss with a consultant. He may want to explore his discomfort when a client cries. He might learn, for instance, that crying is generally a healthy release for clients and that he doesn't need to be concerned about occasional tears or feel that he must cheer up the client. He may also learn that in this case, the client could be showing signs of the kind of depression that needs expert help. A consultant could help him identify those warning signals. Furthermore, Bob could learn some skills in referring a client to a counselor. In this instance, he could let her know that although he is concerned and committed to working with her as her massage therapist, he also wonders if she might want to seek professional counseling to help her get through this difficult time.

When to Use Consultation

Here are some red flags that could indicate you would benefit from a consultation:

- Any strong negative feelings about a client that persist, such as frequently feeling impatient or annoyed with a client, feeling drained by a client, or downright disliking a client.
- Strong positive feelings about a client, wanting to make special exceptions for a client without objective reasons, or wanting to have a sexual relationship with a client.
- Working with a client who is actively dealing with issues of sexual or physical abuse.
- Working with clients who seem unusually depressed or who you suspect might be mentally unbalanced.
- Having trouble setting limits with a particular client.

Supervision

Rather than waiting until they have a problem with a client or are in trouble, many practitioners choose ongoing supervision to gain new awareness and ease in their relationships with clients and to break the isolation of their practices. Supervision can also help when you feel bored with your work.

"Supervision" may sound like someone telling you what to do or how to run your business, and that may make you wary. However, a good supervisor supports and guides, rather than giving unasked-for advice or making you feel inadequate. Time with a supervisor should feel like a visit with a helpful, friendly teacher.

Unlike a consultation, which is generally a one-time or occasional meeting, with supervision, you would get together on a regular basis, perhaps monthly. The goal is to increase your awareness of yourself as a professional and to clarify your strengths and vulnerabilities in the relationship aspect of dealing with clients. (Getting a consultation is a good way to check out how well you would work with a practitioner you are considering for a supervisor.)

Supervision could make your work life more satisfying by helping you understand stumbling blocks that get in your way and by giving you support where you need it, for instance, with setting limits, trusting your intuition, or appreciating your assets. Good supervision can give you confidence and free you up to do your best work.

Good supervision can give you confidence and free you up to do your best work.

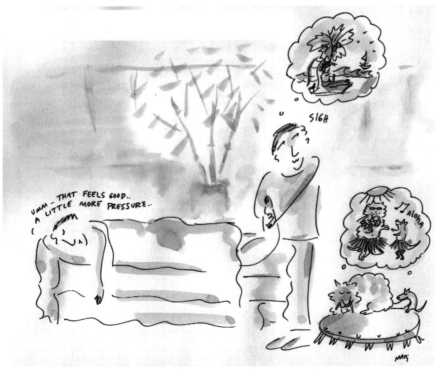

Supervision can help when you feel bored with your work.

A colleague reports:

> At first, I didn't like the idea of supervision, mostly because I was afraid I'd look stupid. After all, I'd been practicing for many years, and I thought I was supposed to have all the answers. However, a friend seemed to be getting so much from her supervision that I decided to try it. To my delight, it was a big boost for my practice. My attitude and behavior toward my clients became more understanding, and clients responded positively to that. The client I had thought was annoying and demanding turned out to be a likable woman who was just frightened about giving up control. The client that I had judged as weird and eccentric turned into a loyal long-term client when I became less judgmental of him. I began to understand my unhelpful patterns and also how to help clients feel more comfortable with me as their practitioner. My practice increased and I was happier with my work life.

When to Use Supervision

You don't need a special reason to seek out supervision. You may just want to grow as a professional, or you may want your practice to be more satisfying. While you would seek out a one-time consultation for a particular client, for instance, you can use supervision when you notice patterns that don't serve you well in your relationships with clients. Here are some red flags that could signal the need for supervision.

- Having a good number of clients who seem "difficult" or controlling
- Having a lot of clients who challenge your boundaries
- Making friends with clients more than once in a blue moon
- Sensing that you "take on" the issues, feelings, or energy of a client in a way that depletes you
- Often feeling sexually attracted to clients
- Frequently feeling drained or exhausted at the end of the day
- Often feeling bored with your work
- Any negative feelings about clients that persist

The Power of Groups

Some practitioners prefer getting together with colleagues, either with or without a supervisor, to share their experiences and knowledge. Some believe that support from colleagues is a must in a profession that is so minimally recognized and acknowledged in the culture. Also, because of the element of touch, somatic practitioners face unique issues that may be understood best by their colleagues.

Many of us have little contact or serious discussion with other manual therapists. I have given workshops in which bodyworkers start a question with, "Maybe I'm the only one this happens to . . . " and then relate a situation that is commonly experienced by practitioners, such as clients being late, clients not giving enough cancellation notice, or clients making sexual advances. It helps to have the reassurance that others are dealing with the same dilemmas.

It also helps to have the validation of talking with a respected colleague or a group of colleagues when you are learning how to set boundaries and limits with your clients. Getting outside support and ideas is fortification for dealing with manipulative or hard-to-handle clients.

Especially in the first years of your practice, you may not know enough to know when you are in over your head or when what a client needs is beyond the scope of your methods or beyond your expertise. You might not fully trust your intuition or recognize a red flag.

Getting together with colleagues in an open, honest, and nonjudgmental environment can be comforting, confidence building, and a boon to your practice. People who stay with this work over the long haul are usually part of a strong group or community of colleagues who support and educate each other.

People who stay with this work over the long haul are usually part of a strong group or community of colleagues who support and educate each other.

GROUP SUPERVISION

Less expensive than individual supervision, group supervision is great for dealing with isolation. It's also a good way for inexperienced practitioners to learn the common issues of this work and gather ideas about the ways others deal with problems that are shared by all practitioners. As with peer support groups, hearing the struggles of others in the group can help you see that you're not alone or unique in the kind of dilemmas that you have. The difference between a peer support group and group supervision is that a supervision group is led by a supervisor and there is usually a fee for attending.

A massage therapist from Seattle praises her supervision group:

> My supervision group has been getting together for a year, meeting every 3 weeks. We alternate meeting with just each other and meeting with a supervisor. Being in the group is helping me move to a place that is healthier with my client relations.
>
> For instance, I've learned that I was brought up to judge my value as a person by how "helpful" and "selfless" I could be. Now I won't work so hard and long on a client that my thumbs are aching, as I used to. I won't take one more client that will be too taxing for my body or mind. I don't take responsibility for clients' healing. I empower them in their healing process. My relationships with my clients feel cleaner with less hidden agendas. And I'm making more money!
>
> I actually went into supervision to learn how to run my business better and make more money. But what was most helpful was that I learned about my boundary problems during the course of being in the group. It's ironic that my initial goals are being met in an entirely roundabout way!

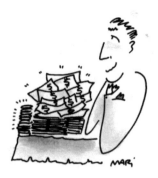

PEER SUPPORT GROUPS

It is possible to meet as a group of practitioners to discuss common issues without a supervisor. Peer groups are not supervised by any of the members and have different benefits than groups that include supervision. Nan Narboe, clinical social worker and boundaries expert, says:

> There are things that only your peers will tell you and that you can only hear from your peers. For instance, if our supervisor praises a piece of work we do, we may assume she's "just being nice." If we hear the same praise from our peers, we tend to believe it. There are times, however, when individual supervision is best. There are things that only your supervisor will tell you and that you can only hear from your supervisor, such as where your blind spots are.

Peer groups are an excellent and inexpensive way to get support and learn from others. Groups may also want to hire a consultant to work with them occasionally on a specific issue or for a specific purpose.

Jack Blackburn, LMP, certified Trager practitioner, registered counselor, and supervisor for bodyworkers, reinforces the need for meeting with colleagues: "The main reason practitioners burn out isn't because they work too hard or take too much responsibility for their clients. It's because they don't have a place to talk with other massage therapists and bodyworkers about what happens in their practices." Blackburn teaches practitioners how to support their peers, in addition to professional supervision, using active listening and other processes to help each other understand their relationships with clients.

Benefits of Supervision and Consultation

Here are some of the reasons that consultations and supervision, whether in a group or individually, are invaluable to both inexperienced and seasoned practitioners.

Identifying Blind Spots

We all have less than positive ways of interacting that we tend to put out of our awareness—ways that we might unconsciously hurt clients, ways that we might overstep boundaries. We need feedback from someone who has the skill and willingness to tell us what we do not see about ourselves. Our teachers don't always do this, nor do all friends, partners, or spouses. We like to think of ourselves as always caring, and it can be painful to have someone, even diplomatically, point out ways we might be insensitive to others. But how else are we going to learn?

Ethics consultant Daphne Chellos says it straight out:

> Supervision is a preventive measure against abusing clients. Abuse can be unintentional as well as intentional, subtle as well as blatant. As humans, all of us can be "victims" and all of us can be "aggressors." Our tendency is to remember violations against us and to either forget or ignore our aggressive acts. This blind spot exists as well in therapeutic relationships. A competent supervisor will notice when a therapist is being inappropriate or abusive, no matter how subtly or unintentionally, and bring it to the therapist's attention.[1]

"Abuse" may seem like a strong word. It is used here to mean anything a practitioner does that could, even in a minor way, take advantage of or wound a client—from an insensitive remark about the client's body to overcharging for services.

Keeping Confidentiality

Clients tell us their secrets. Even if they don't tell us, we might guess. Perhaps we realize how frightened that successful, confident-looking businessman actually is because we see the tension in his body. Maybe we sense the underlying sadness of the vivacious woman who tries so hard to be upbeat. Clients confide in us about their private lives and concerns, but as professionals, we're not allowed to talk about our clients with our colleagues, friends, or families, and we're certainly not allowed to divulge anything they say. As Trager instructor Amrita Daigle says, "If we don't have someone who we can talk with in professional confidence, we will tend to gossip about our clients." It can become a burden to carry all that pain, all those secrets. Having a supervisor who is also bound by rules of confidentiality gives us a way to share that burden.

---

[1]Chellos D. Supervision in bodywork: Borrowing a model from psychotherapy. Massage Therapy Journal 1991;Winter;30:15.

Easing Guilt

I've talked with many practitioners who feel ashamed of an instance when they used poor judgment or went outside professional boundaries. Sometimes no harm was done to the client, and sometimes the practitioner couldn't have foreseen the problem. However, these moments weigh on practitioners who strive to be ethical. Talking with a trusted supervisor or mentor helps put those mistakes in perspective. A good supervisor will hear our mistakes and errors without making us feel ashamed or incompetent.

Recognizing Prejudice

How do we really feel about working with other races, gays and lesbians, overweight people, the chronically ill, racists, Orthodox Jews, Hindus, Muslims, born-again Christians—just to name a few groups? What about people who voted for the candidate we campaigned against? Or sexist men, pampered women, angry feminists? Do any of these types of people make our hearts snap shut? Everyone makes prejudgments to some degree. Supervision helps us recognize these prejudgments so that we can either get beyond our negative feelings and learn to either care about the client or refer the client to someone else.

Getting Help With Mentally Ill Clients

We will probably encounter emotionally disturbed people in our practices, and they will respond to us and our work differently than will other clients. We may be baffled by their behavior or insensitive to their fears. Or we may not know how to take care of ourselves when we are working with them. A supervisor trained in psychological dynamics is a valuable resource for helping us identify and figure out what to do with clients who may be mentally ill.

Clients with mental illness can make complaints or feel harmed even when practitioners are ethical and careful. As caring practitioners, we may want to help a client who appears to be floundering. Yet some people who are mentally ill can exhibit extreme helplessness on the one hand and rage on the other. We may be ill-fatedly drawn to try to rescue a seemingly helpless client, only to wind up as the recipient of that person's anger. For our own protection, we need help identifying mental illness.

Although it is not our place to make a specific diagnosis, we do want to know whether a client is mentally ill for his or her protection as well as our own. For example, people with a mental illness generally don't have the interior strength to weather a process that can strip away defenses, such as emotionally oriented work. Ordinary folks seek out that kind of work in order to experience a deeper part of themselves. For disturbed people, who may feel blank or chaotic behind their social exterior, such work can be uncomfortable and disorienting. An experienced supervisor can help us identify signs of mental illness and judge whether our work will be beneficial to the prospective client. Of course, if the client is being treated by a mental health professional, we should ask the client for permission to speak with him or her to find out whether our work will be helpful to the client.

Supporting Our Intuition

Many manual therapists use their intuition to understand how best to work with clients. Intuition is a useful gift, but sometimes it fails us. Sometimes clients slip beneath the radar of our intuition, or we need more information to be able to understand them. We may misread them and fail to offer the kind of support they need. A good supervisor could help us see the reasons we didn't understand the client and educate us about how best to use our intuitive side.

And the #1 Reason for Getting Supervision

Perhaps it's a little late to say this, but good boundaries can't be entirely learned from reading a book. We have to experience them. We need to experience the safety of working with someone who is clear and careful with boundaries. We have to get the solid feeling of good boundaries inside us.

A book can give us an idea of why it's important to be professional, but we can't learn it all from a book. Many of us have had a few teachers along the way who were careless or uneducated about relationship issues, and we need a remedial experience. If we aspire to a high level of professionalism, we need the good modeling that a compassionate professional trained in transference and countertransference can provide.

Finding Help and Support

For manual therapists, getting help with the relationship aspect of our work or coming together to support each other are still new concepts. Certainly practitioners get together informally with friends who are also bodyworkers to encourage each other and talk about common issues. However, more organized ways of meeting together are still not that widely practiced. But casual sharing, aside from the possibility of leading to violations of confidentiality, doesn't always offer the depth of support and insight that we need. Fortunately, practitioners can now find and create other ways to enrich their professional lives.

Choosing a Consultant or Supervisor

Because getting consultations and supervision for the relationship issues of this work is a fairly new idea, you will have to be creative in finding someone with whom to work. The practitioner you choose should be someone who is trained in psychological dynamics and appreciates bodywork and massage. A psychiatric social worker, psychologist, or other mental health professional who has never experienced bodywork may not be able to understand the intimacy of the work and the problems involved. Your consultant or supervisor should also respect the profession and be aware that manual therapists perform a valuable service for the community.

You can also work with a bodyworker or massage therapist who has training and experience in relationship dynamics. Although that would be ideal, few manual practitioners have such training.

There is no set way to find someone who will suit you. You can ask others for the names of good psychotherapists in your community and see if they would be interested in working with you. They have to understand that you don't want personal counseling, and they need to know the difference between consulting about work issues and doing psychotherapy. Not all psychotherapists have the experience or the inclination to do this kind of consulting.

Because you are hoping to learn more about good relationship boundaries, it should be obvious that your consultant or supervisor needs to be someone with whom you don't have another relationship.

Keep in mind that because the consultant or supervisor doesn't need to see your hands-on work, supervision and consultation can occur by phone. If you live in a small town, you may choose to have telephone appointments with an out-of-town consultant who does not know you or your clients.

You want someone who gives you the feeling that you have a new ally, that you have someone in your corner.

When you are trying out a supervisor or consultant, you want to notice if this is someone who helps you trust your own intuition, who can suggest new choices without making you feel judged, who is enthusiastic about your work, and who helps you feel more confident. You want someone who gives you the feeling that you have a new ally, that you have someone in your corner.

Forming a Peer Group

While in school, many students form close bonds with other students but do not keep in touch once they have graduated. Once out in their practices, massage therapists and bodyworkers don't always have an awareness of how crucial it is to their professional health to stay in touch with colleagues.

To start a group, you have to round up some colleagues who would like to get together regularly to share experiences. An ideal number would be between four and 12 participants. It's a good idea to ask members to commit to meeting on a regular schedule for a certain length of time—perhaps once or twice a month for at least 6 meetings—to give the group a chance to gel.

Groups need to adhere to rules of confidentiality in agreeing not to talk outside the group about what other members say there. Also, members should agree to make every effort to disguise the identity of clients they are discussing.

It's a good idea if group members agree to other ground rules as well, such as not offering advice unless they are asked or not interrupting others. Care should be taken to give each member a chance to bring their issues to the group. Although a small amount of venting can be useful, groups shouldn't be allowed to deteriorate into gripe sessions.

It's important that groups state their intentions clearly from the beginning, for instance, that they're interested in learning from each other and wanting to grow as professionals.

A Word About Mentoring

With mentoring, you make an agreement with a more experienced colleague that she or he will be available to answer your questions. It can be an informal arrangement and is often unpaid. It may be as simple as, "Let me take you to lunch and get the benefit of your years as a bodyworker." Everyone graduating from manual therapy training needs mentors. It should be a given that you're not expected to start a practice without help and support.

Mentoring usually addresses less complex issues than supervision addresses. It's good for business and practice-building kinds of questions, such as the value of using an answering service or the pros and cons of working out of your home.

A mentor can be any practitioner you respect whose work is similar to yours and who is willing to meet with you to share his or her experiences.

These days, it's even possible to find excellent mentoring on an online forum for massage therapists or bodyworkers. On such forums, there are hundreds of massage therapists and bodyworkers with varying levels of experience. Participants can ask questions that they would ask a mentor and receive a wide range of advice. The obvious disadvantage of this method is that there isn't the face-to-face relationship that can provide more personal encouragement and support, and you don't necessarily know the qualifications of the people responding.

Taking Care of Ourselves

To forestall burnout, somatic practitioners need to learn how to take good care of themselves, which means getting help from others. Sharing with someone else what really goes on in our offices, what pushes our buttons, and where our hearts get shut down is crucial to the health of our practices.

The work we do is complex and demanding. Consultations, supervision, peer support, and mentoring can take away the isolation and depletion that can kill our interest in our work. Our professional lives are more rewarding when we find ways to keep our interest alive and be kinder to ourselves.

QUESTIONS FOR REFLECTION

1. If you are a student, what steps can you take when you finish your training to make sure you have the support and information you need? If you are already practicing, do you have enough support to keep you excited and encouraged about your work? Do you have any resources to help you sort out the therapeutic relationship aspect of your work? What steps could you take to make sure you have enough support and resources?

2. How do you feel about the idea of going to someone for supervision or consultation? What would be the pros and cons for you personally?

3. Are there areas where you could benefit from help—for instance, setting limits, working with women who have been sexually abused, or knowing how to work with an emotionally fragile client? What are the areas that are the most challenging for you? What can you do to help you feel more confident about these areas?

4. If you are already practicing, can you think of a time when a problem with a client would have gone more smoothly if you had had outside professional help with it? How would you handle that situation now?

Appendix A

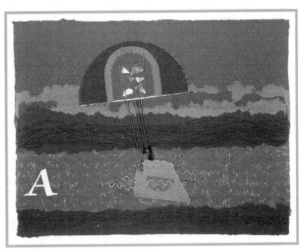

AMERICAN MASSAGE THERAPY ASSOCIATION CODE OF ETHICS[1]

This Code of Ethics is a summary statement of the standards by which massage therapists agree to conduct their practices and is a declaration of the general principles of acceptable, ethical, professional behavior.

Massage therapists shall:

1. Demonstrate commitment to provide the highest quality massage therapy/bodywork to those who seek their professional service.

2. Acknowledge the inherent worth and individuality of each person by not discriminating or behaving in any prejudicial manner with clients and/or colleagues.

3. Demonstrate professional excellence through regular self-assessment of strengths, limitations, and effectiveness by continued education and training.

4. Acknowledge the confidential nature of the professional relationship with clients and respect each client's right to privacy.

5. Conduct all business and professional activities within their scope of practice, the law of the land, and project a professional image.

6. Refrain from engaging in any sexual conduct or sexual activities involving their clients.

7. Accept responsibility to do no harm to the physical, mental and emotional well-being of self, clients, and associates.

[1]Used with permission of American Massage Therapy Association, ©2001. For information on joining AMTA, call 847/864-0123.

Appendix **B**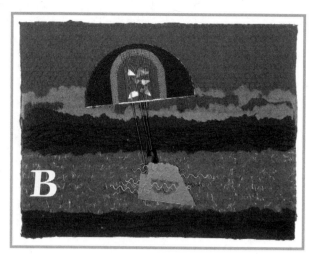

$\mathcal{A}$SSOCIATED BODYWORK AND MASSAGE PROFESSIONALS CODE OF ETHICS[1]

As a member of Associated Bodywork & Massage Professionals, I hereby pledge to abide by the ABMP Code of Ethics as outlined below.

Client Relationships

- I shall endeavor to serve the best interests of my clients at all times and to provide the highest quality service possible.
- I shall maintain clear and honest communications with my clients and shall keep client communications confidential.
- I shall acknowledge the limitations of my skills and, when necessary, refer clients to the appropriate qualified health care professional.
- I shall in no way instigate or tolerate any kind of sexual advance while acting in the capacity of a massage, bodywork, somatic therapy or esthetic practitioner.

---

[1]Courtesy of Associated Bodywork & Massage Professionals. For information on membership, call 800-458-2267 or visit www.abmp.com.

Professionalism

- I shall maintain the highest standards of professional conduct, providing services in an ethical and professional manner in relation to my clientele, business associates, health care professionals, and the general public.
- I shall respect the rights of all ethical practitioners and will cooperate with all health care professionals in a friendly and professional manner.
- I shall refrain from the use of any mind-altering drugs, alcohol, or intoxicants prior to or during professional sessions.
- I shall always dress in a professional manner, proper dress being defined as attire suitable and consistent with accepted business and professional practice.
- I shall not be affiliated with or employed by any business that utilizes any form of sexual suggestiveness or explicit sexuality in its advertising or promotion of services, or in the actual practice of its services.

Scope of Practice/Appropriate Techniques

- I shall provide services within the scope of the ABMP definition of massage, bodywork, somatic therapies and skin care, and the limits of my training. I will not employ those massage, bodywork or skin care techniques for which I have not had adequate training and shall represent my education, training, qualifications and abilities honestly.
- I shall be conscious of the intent of the services that I am providing and shall be aware of and practice good judgment regarding the application of massage, bodywork or somatic techniques utilized.
- I shall not perform manipulations or adjustments of the human skeletal structure, diagnose, prescribe or provide any other service, procedure or therapy which requires a license to practice chiropractic, osteopathy, physical therapy, podiatry, orthopedics, psychotherapy, acupuncture, dermatology, cosmetology, or any other profession or branch of medicine unless specifically licensed to do so.
- I shall be thoroughly educated and understand the physiological effects of the specific massage, bodywork, somatic or skin care techniques utilized in order to determine whether such application is contraindicated and/or to determine the most beneficial techniques to apply to a given individual. I shall not apply massage, bodywork, somatic or skin care techniques in those cases where they may be contraindicated without a written referral from the client's primary care provider.

Image/Advertising Claims

- I shall strive to project a professional image for myself, my business or place of employment, and the profession in general.
- I shall actively participate in educating the public regarding the actual benefits of massage, bodywork, somatic therapies and skin care.
- I shall practice honesty in advertising, promote my services ethically and in good taste, and practice and/or advertise only those techniques for which I have received adequate training and/or certification. I shall not make false claims regarding the potential benefits of the techniques rendered.

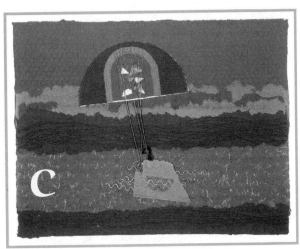

Appendix C

*R*ELATED READINGS

Benjamin BE, Sohnen-Moe CM. The Ethics of Touch. Tucson, AZ: Sohnen-Moe Associates, 2003.

Berne E. Games People Play: The Basic Handbook of Transactional Analysis. New York: Ballantine, 1996.

Borysenko J. Minding the Body, Mending the Mind. New York: Bantam Press, 1988.

Cousins N. The Healing Heart. New York: WW Norton, 1983.

Dychtwald K. Body-Mind. New York: Jeremy P. Tarcher, 1986.

Fanning P, McKay M, Davis M. Messages: The Communication Skills Book, 2nd ed. Oakland, CA: New Harbinger Publications, 1995.

Ford CW. Compassionate Touch: The Body's Role in Emotional Healing and Recovery. Berkeley, CA: North Atlantic Books, 1999.

Frank JD, Frank JB. Persuasion and Healing. Baltimore: Johns Hopkins University Press, 1993.

Fritz S. Mosby's Fundamentals of Therapeutic Massage, 2nd ed. St. Louis: Mosby, 2000.

Greene E, Goodrich-Dunn B. The Psychology of the Body. Baltimore: Lippincott, Williams & Wilkins, 2003.

Herman JL. Trauma and Recovery. New York: Harper Collins Publishers, 1992.

Johnson DH, ed. Bone, Breath, and Gesture: Practices of Embodiment. Berkeley, CA: North Atlantic Books, 1995.

Juhan D. Job's Body: A Handbook for Bodywork, 3rd ed. Barrytown, NY: Barrytown Ltd., 2003.

Keleman S. Emotional Anatomy. Berkeley, CA: Center Press, 1985.

Kurtz R. Body-Centered Psychotherapy, The Hakomi Method. Mendocino, CA: LifeRhythm Press, 1990.

Levine PA. Waking the Tiger-Healing Trauma. Berkeley, CA: North Atlantic Books, 1997.

Naparstek B. Invisible Heroes: Survivors of Trauma and How They Heal. New York: Bantam, 2004.

Narboe N. Working With What You Can't Get Your Hands On. Portland, OR: Narboe, 1985.

Pert CB. Molecules of Emotion. New York: Touchstone, Simon & Schuster, 1997.

Rosen M, Brenner S. Rosen Method Bodywork: Accessing the Unconscious through Touch. Berkeley, CA: North Atlantic Books, 2003.

Rothschild B. The Body Remembers: The Psychophysiology of Trauma and Trauma Treatment. New York: WW Norton, 2000.

Scaer R. The Body Bears the Burden: Trauma, Dissociation, and Disease. Binghamton, NY: Haworth Press, 2001.

Smith FF. Inner Bridges: A Guide to Energy Movement and Body Structure. Atlanta: Humanics New Age, 1986.

Sohnen-Moe CM. Business Mastery. Tucson, AZ. Sohnen-Moe Associates, 1997.

Taylor K. The Ethics of Caring: Honoring the Web of Life in Our Professional Healing Relationships. Santa Cruz, CA: Hanford Mead, 1995.

Thompson DL. Hands Heal: Communication, Documentation, and Insurance Billing for Manual Therapists, 2nd ed. Baltimore: Lippincott, Williams & Wilkins, 2001.

Wooten S. Touching the Body, Reaching the Soul. Santa Fe, NM: Wooten, 1995.

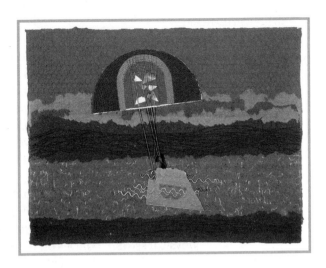

GLOSSARY

Alexander technique: A re-education of the mind and body that intends to change movement habits in everyday activities. It aims to release tension and improve ease and freedom of movement, balance, support, and coordination. Developed by F. M. Alexander

Altered state: A state of consciousness in which we are more deeply relaxed, less aware of our thinking minds, and more open and vulnerable than we are in our day-to-day functioning.

Bartering: Used here to mean exchanging a manual therapy session for goods or services other than another manual therapy session.

Boundaries: In this context, a boundary is like a protective circle around the professional relationship that separates what is appropriate between practitioner and client from what is not. Keeping appropriate boundaries includes such behavior as not engaging a client in another kind of relationship, such as a social one, and honoring what is appropriate within the professional relationship, such as confidentiality.

Consultation: A meeting with a professional trained in psychological dynamics to obtain advice and insight about a particular client or issue.

Contract: An agreement between practitioner and client that is often implied rather than explicit about what each will or will not do. An ethical contract must be within the bounds of the practitioner's training and the ethical standards of her or his profession. The client agrees to give specific fees, goods, or services in return and agrees to be respectful of the practitioner's guidelines for appropriate behavior.

Countertransference: When a practitioner allows unresolved feelings and personal issues to influence his relationship with a client.

Dual relationship: Having a relationship with a client other than the contractual therapeutic one, such as having a client who is also a friend, family member, or business associate.

Emotionally oriented bodywork: Manual therapy that is based on the idea that physical tension and restriction are related to unconscious patterns of holding that the client has adopted, often early in life, to cope with his or her emotional environment. The practitioner facilitates the client in releasing these tension patterns for the greater emotional and physical well-being of the client. Also called *psychologically oriented bodywork.*

Feldenkrais Method: A movement therapy that seeks to re-educate the body and mind through movements that tap into the nervous system's own innate processes to change and refine functioning. Developed by Moshe Feldenkrais.

Framework: The logistics by which practitioners define themselves as professional and create a safe atmosphere for clients. Framework includes the ways that we present ourselves in advertising, the preparation of the physical setting, policies on fees and time, and such ground rules as keeping the focus on the client.

Healing Touch: A holistic energy therapy that uses gentle, noninvasive touch to influence and support the human energy system within and surrounding the body. The goal of Healing Touch is to restore harmony, energy, and balance within the human energy system.

Informed consent: The client's authorization for services to be performed by the practitioner. The client or the client's guardian must be fully advised of what the service will entail and its benefits and any contraindications and must be competent to give consent.

Manual therapists: Trained professionals who touch the physical or energetic body of the client or who use a method of movement to affect the body of a client for the purpose of facilitating awareness, health, and well-being. The term as used here is interchangeable with *somatic practitioners* and includes massage therapists, bodyworkers, movement educators, practitioners of Oriental methods, and practitioners who work primarily with energy fields.

Mentor: A trusted colleague who provides guidance and education. Mentors are usually helpful in advising on both the details of establishing oneself as a professional and the broader general aspects of taking on a professional role or of taking on the role of a particular kind of bodywork or massage practitioner.

Peer group: A group of colleagues who meet regularly to discuss common issues related to their professional lives, to share information and strategies, and to receive emotional support.

Polarity therapy: In the bodywork part of this therapy, the practitioner works with the client's energy field—electromagnetic patterns expressed in mental, emotional, and physical experience—to facilitate greater health. Developed by Dr. Randolph Stone.

Posttraumatic stress disorder (PTSD): A type of anxiety disorder that can develop after experiencing a very traumatic or life-threatening event. It can cause flashbacks; sleep problems; nightmares; hypervigilance; feelings of isolation, guilt, and paranoia; and sometimes panic attacks.

Professional therapeutic relationship: A relationship between client and practitioner that is focused on the well-being of the client and is contractual.

Reiki: A form of energy healing. Reiki involves gentle touch that directs chi for the purpose of strengthening the client's energy system. *Chi* is the term used by Chinese mystics and martial artists for universal life energy.

Right of refusal: The entitlement of both the client and the practitioner to end a session or to decline to receive or give a particular kind of manipulation or technique.

Role-playing: Usually a structured exercise in which students or colleagues take a role—for instance, as client or practitioner—and act out a specific situation as a way of becoming more comfortable with handling the situation in real life.

Rolfing: Manipulation of the myofascial system to integrate the physical structure toward greater balance, ease, and centeredness by releasing tension patterns in the connective tissue. Developed by Dr. Ida P. Rolf.

Rosen Method bodywork: A method that uses gentle touch coupled with verbal communication to help clients become aware of and release unconscious physical and emotional tension. The practitioner notices changes in muscle tension and shifts in breathing patterns and uses them as a guide to enhance clients' awareness of their internal experience. Developed by Marion Rosen.

Rubenfeld Synergy Method: A holistic therapy that uses gentle touch along with verbal dialogue, active listening, Gestalt Process, imagery, metaphor, movement, and humor. It is based on the belief that unacknowledged feelings from past experiences are stored in our bodies and unconsciously affect our behavior, attitudes, and self-image. This method has the intention of allowing buried feelings and memories to surface, freeing clients from old patterns and energy blocks. Developed by Ilana Rubenfeld.

Somatic practitioners: Trained professionals who touch the physical or energetic body of the client or who use a method of movement to affect the body of a client for the purpose of facilitating awareness, health, and well-being. The term as used here is interchangeable with *manual therapists* and includes massage therapists, bodyworkers, movement educators, practitioners of Oriental methods, and practitioners who work primarily with energy fields.

Supervision: An ongoing arrangement made with a professional trained in psychological dynamics for help with the relationship aspects of a practitioner's work. Supervision includes clarifying the practitioner's countertransference issues, suggesting effective interventions and identifying the practitioner's vulnerabilities and areas of strength.

Trager Approach: Hands-on movement education that uses gentle movements to release physical and emotional tension patterns and facilitate relaxation, increased physical mobility, and mental clarity. Created and developed by Dr. Milton Trager.

Transference: When a client unconsciously projects (transfers) unresolved feelings, needs, and issues—usually from childhood and usually related to parent or other authority figures—onto a practitioner.

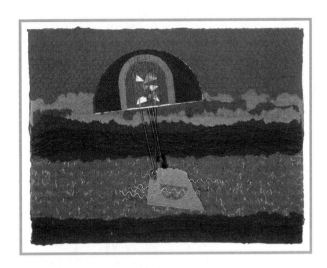

INDEX

A

Advertising, 28, 116–117
Alexander technique, 179
Altered state, communication and, 84
American Massage Therapy Association Code of Ethics, 173
Answering machines, 28–30
Appearance, professional, 110
Appointments
  missed, 139–141
  scheduling of, 30, 35–36
Assault, prevention of, 117–118
Associated Bodywork and Massage Professionals Code of Ethics, 174–176
Attire, professional, 110

B

Bartering
  complications of, 152–154
  definition of, 147
  dual relationships and, 147, 152–154
    (*see also* Dual relationships)
  financial boundaries and, 106
  transference and, 106
Bauer, Rob, 30, 156
Blackburn, Jack, 166
Blind spots, identification of, 167
Body image, 88, 90
Body jewelry, 110

Bodywork (*see* Deep structural bodywork; Emotionally oriented bodywork)
Bodyworkers (*see* Manual therapists)
Boundaries, professional (*see* Professional boundaries)
Breasts, working near, 112
Brenneke, Heida, 112
Business cards, 27–28, 116–117
Business coaches, 144–145
Business relationships, 72–73, 154–155
Business transactions, 23
Businesses, outside, 23, 72–73, 154–155

C

Captive audience, transference and, 54–55
Chellos, Daphne, 167
Chronic complainers, response to, 67–68, 81–82
Chronic pain, 42
Cleanliness, of work space, 32–33
Client-practitioner dynamics, 46–63 (*see also* Therapeutic relationship)
  countertransference and, 50–52, 58–63
  transference and, 46–58
Client(s)
  abrupt termination of therapy by, 42–43

Client(s) *(continued)*
advice-seeking, 92
caretaking by, 40
in chronic pain, 42
communication with (*see* Communication)
complaints of, response to, 67–68, 80–81, 141–142
demanding, 95–96
dependent, 55
disrespectful, 15, 73–75, 118–119
draping of, 33, 111
emotional, 92–93
emotionally disturbed, 41, 105, 125–126, 155–156, 168–169
expectations of, 34
former, dating relationship with, 69–70, 104–106
frameworks for, 40–42
as friends, 17–18, 37, 66–67, 69–70, 103, 148–150
friends as, 150–152
gifts from, 143
informed consent of, 15, 34, 78–79
initial phone contact with, 30–31 (*see also* Telephone calls)
interaction among, 39–40
needs of, 9
negative feelings toward, 70–72, 167, 168
new, 30–31, 40–41
passive, 53–54
personal questions by, 94–95
privacy rights of, 14, 29, 36, 37–39, 66, 75–76 (*see also* Confidentiality)
referrals by, 76, 143–144
referrals for, 61, 72
refusal to treat, 15, 73–74
relationship with (*see* Therapeutic relationship)
relatives as, 150–152
respect for, 67–68
right of refusal of, 15, 34
romantic/sexual attraction and, 18, 55–56, 59, 61, 66–67, 101–103
safety of, 2–3
screening of, 117
seductive, 125–126

sex-seeking, 115–123
sexually abused, 41–42, 107–110, 112
socialization with, 17–18, 37, 66–67, 69–70, 103, 148–152
talkative, 91–92
tips from, 142–143
traumatized, 41–42, 107–110, 112
Clothing
client, 111
practitioner, 110
Coaches, 144–145 (*see also* Consultation; Mentoring; Supervision)
Coccyx, working near, 112
Codes of ethics, 173–176
Colleagues, support from, 164–166, 170–171
Commercial transactions, 23
Common sense, versus professional boundaries, 6–7
Communication, 84–98
about boundaries, 96–98
about fees, 134–135
after abrupt termination of therapy, 41–42
altered state and, 84
common dilemmas in, 91–96
countertransference and, 85–86
with demanding clients, 95–96
guidelines for, 87–91
by instant messaging, 37
outside of office, 37
personal questions by clients and, 94–95
positive versus negative messages in, 84–85
role playing and, 98
scope of practice and, 95
during sessions, 87–91
sexual boundaries and, 111
with talkative clients, 91–92
by telephone, 28–31 (*see also* Telephone calls)
transference and, 84
Complaints
about sexual boundary violations, 124, 128–129
refunds and, 141–142
response to, 67–68, 80–81
Confidentiality, 14, 36, 37–39, 66, 75–77, 167

dual relationships and, 157
   peer groups and, 170
   of phone messages, 29
Consent, 15, 34, 78–79
Consistency, in therapeutic relationship, 14–15
Consultation, 161–162
   about countertransference, 61–62, 126
   about transference, 102–103
   benefits of, 77, 161–162, 167–169
   definition of, 161
   examples of, 161–162
   getting started with, 169–170
   versus supervision, 163 (*see also* Supervision)
   when to use, 162
Contract, therapeutic, 12
Control issues, in therapeutic relationship, 86–87
Counseling, 8, 20–22, 75
   for countertransference, 61–62
   by practitioner, 8, 20–22, 75, 92
   referral for, 75, 93–94
   for sexually abused clients, 108
Countertransference, 50–52, 58–63
   (*see also* Transference)
   communication and, 85–86
   consultation for, 61–62, 126
   dealing with, 60–62
   definition of, 51
   negative, 59–60
   positive, 59, 103–104
   seductive patients and, 125–126
   signs of, 58–60, 61, 125–126
   transference and, 51–52
Crushes, 55–56, 101–103 (*see also* Sexual boundaries)
Crying, 93

D
Daigle, Amrita, 77, 167
Dating (*see also* Sexual boundaries)
   of ex-clients, 69–70, 104–105
Deep structural bodywork
   framework for, 41
   transference and, 105–106
Demanding clients, 95–96
Demonstrations, 28
Dependency, transference and, 55

Discounts, 82, 136–139
Disrespectful clients, 15, 73–75, 118–119
Disrobing, 111
Documentation, legal aspects of, 82
Draping, 33, 111
Dual relationships, 106, 146–159
   bartering/trading and, 146–147, 152–154
   business relationships and, 72–73, 154–155
   common problems in, 147–155
   confidentiality and, 157
   definition of, 146
   dynamics of, 146–147
   guidelines for, 155–158
   product sales and, 23, 72–73, 154–155
   students and, 157–158
   transference and, 155–156

E
Early arrivals, 34–35
Electronic medical records, privacy of, 38
Emotionally disturbed clients
   dual relationships and, 155–156
   framework for, 41
   help with, 168–169
   sexual boundaries and, 125–126
   transference and, 105
Emotionally oriented bodywork
   definition of, 105
   dual relationships and, 156
   framework for, 41
   transference and, 105–106
Emotions, uncovering of, 3
Erections, dealing with, 120–123
Ethical boundaries
   client dignity and, 67–68
   client vulnerability and, 65
   codes of ethics and, 173–176
   impropriety and, 66–67
   judgment calls and, 67–77
   legal aspects of, 80–83
   purpose of, 65
   self-assessment for, 64–65
   sexual issues and, 123–127 (*see also* Sexual boundaries)
   supervision and, 167
   violation of, 65–66, 168

Ethical decision-making, 67–77
Ethical issues
  confidentiality, 14, 29, 65
  examples of, 67–77
  false claims, 77
  financial gain, 72–73
  negative feelings toward client, 70–72
  outside businesses, 23
  privacy and confidentiality, 14, 29,
    36, 37–39, 66, 75–77, 157,
    167, 170
  romantic/sexual feelings, 18, 55–56,
    59, 61, 66–70, 101–106
  scope of practice, 78
Ex-clients, dating relationship with,
    69–70, 104–106
Expertise, scope of, 19

F
Family members, as clients, 150–152
Fees, 135–139 (*see also* Financial
    boundaries)
  discounted, 82, 136–139
  for missed appointments, 139–141
  raising, 136
  setting, 135
Feldenkrais Method, 180
Financial boundaries, 131–145
  comfort level with, 144–145
  communication and, 134–135
  emotional aspects of, 133–134
  fee policies and, 135–139 (*see also* Fees)
  gift certificates and, 141
  gifts and, 143
  gratuities and, 142–143
  kickbacks and, 144
  mentors and, 144–145
  missed appointments and, 139–141
  practitioner discomfort with, 132
  profit versus caring and, 131–132
  refunds and, 141–142
  rewards for referrals and, 143–144
  setting limits and, 134–135
  therapeutic relationship and, 131–132
  workshops for, 144–145
Financial gain, ethical aspects of, 72–73
Flirting (*see* Romantic feelings)
Former clients, dating relationship
    with, 69–70, 104–106
Framework(s), 25–45

  advertising and, 26–30
  for basic session, 33–40 (*see also*
    Therapy sessions)
  bending of, 43–44
  benefits of, 44–45
  for deep emotional work, 41
  definition of, 25
  inattention to, 26–27
  initial client contact and, 30–31
  need for, 26–27
  for regular clients, 40–41
  self-presentation and, 26–31
  for specific types of clients, 40–41
  for structural bodywork, 41
  telephone calls and, 28–31
  therapeutic setting and, 31–33
Frank, Jerome, 132
Friend(s)
  as clients, 150–152
  clients as, 17–18, 37, 66–67, 69–70,
    103, 148–150 (*see also* Dual
    relationships)
Fritz, Sandy, 23

G
Gender dynamics, 126–127
Genital area, working near, 112
Gift certificates, 141
Gifts, from clients, 143
Glossary of terms, 179–181
Group supervision, 165

H
Healing touch, 180
Health records, privacy of, 38
Health-related products, sale of, 23,
    72–73, 154–155
Home offices, 30–32 (*see also* Work
    space)
Hugging, 112
Hygiene, client, 73–74

I
Informed consent, 15, 34, 78–79
Insecurity, professional, 19–20
Instant messaging, 37
Internet
  advertising on, 28
  instant messaging and, 37
  privacy and, 38
Intuition, 169

K

Kertay, Les, 43
Kickbacks, 144

L

Late arrivals, 34–35
Legal issues, 80–83 (*see also* Ethical boundaries; Ethical issues)
  informed consent, 15, 34, 78–79
  reporting of sexual boundary violations, 129
  right of refusal, 15, 34, 73–74
Liben, Lucy, 112
Locked doors, sexual boundaries and, 111
Lost souls, 55

M

Male clients, erections in, 120–123
Malpractice, 80–83
Manual therapists (*see also* Somatic practitioners; *under terms beginning with* Professional)
  clients of (*see* Client(s))
  definition of, 1, 180
  denigration of by other practitioners, 80
  excessive talking by, 17–18
  medical advice from, 20
  mistaken for sex workers, 115–119 (*see also* Sexual boundaries)
  personal needs of, 40
  practice termination by, 43
  professional appearance of, 110
  professional associations for, 82
  professional rights of, 15
  professional roles of, 12–13
  psychological advice from, 20–22
  relocation of, 43
  right of refusal of, 15, 73
  self-care for, 171
  sexually predatory behavior by, 127–130
  spiritual advice by, 22–23
  support for, 160–171
Manual therapy
  false claims about, 77
  overview of, 1
  professional boundaries in (*see* Professional boundaries)
  professional relationship in, 12–24 (*see also* Therapeutic relationship)
  termination of
    by client, 42–43
    by therapist, 43
Masturbation, during therapy session, 119
Medical advice, 20
Medical records, privacy of, 38
Mentally ill clients
  dual relationships and, 155–156
  framework for, 41
  help with, 168–169
  sexual boundaries and, 125–126
  transference and, 105
Mentoring, 144–145, 171
Missed appointments, 139–141
Money matters (*see* Fees; Financial boundaries)

N

Name-dropping, 76
Narboe, Nan, 72, 166
Negative feelings, toward clients, 70–72, 167, 168
New clients
  framework for, 40–41
  telephone contact with, 30–31
Nutritional supplements, sale of, 23, 72–73, 154–155

O

Office (*see* Work space)
Outcalls, 117–118
Outside businesses, 23, 72–73, 154–155

P

Pain, chronic, 42
Peer support, 164–166, 170–171
Personal hygiene, of client, 73–74
Personal information
  communication of by client, 20–22
  communication of by therapist, 17–18 (*see also* Confidentiality)
Personal questions, by clients, 94–95
Personal versus professional needs, 8–9
Phillips, Lee, 118–119
Phone calls (*see* Telephone calls)
Physical affection, 112

Piercings, 110
Polarity therapy, 180
Polseno, Dianne, 157–158
Power
 barriers and, 5
 responsibility and, 4
 in therapeutic relationship, 86–87
 transference and, 53–54, 58
Practice (*see also* Manual therapy)
 closing of, 43
Practitioners (*see* Manual therapists)
Prejudice, recognition of, 168
Privacy issues, 14, 29, 36, 37–39, 66,
  75–77 (*see also* Confidentiality)
Product sales, 23, 72–73, 154–155
Professional appearance, 110
Professional associations, membership
  in, 82
Professional boundaries, 12–13
 artificiality of, 6–7
 as barriers, 5–6, 23–24
 bending of, 43–44
 client-practitioner dynamics and,
  46–63
 communication of, 96–98
 countertransference and, 58–63
 definition of, 2
 dual relationships and, 146–159
 establishment of, 96–98
 excluded elements in, 16–23
 financial, 131–145
 framework for, 25–45
 help with, 160–172 (*see also* Consultation; Supervision)
 inattention to, 9–10
 included elements in, 12–15
 as just common sense, 6–7
 misconceptions about, 4–10
 need for, 2–4
 outside business ventures and, 23,
  72–73, 154–155
 power and, 5
 as protective circles, 12–24 (*see also*
  Therapeutic relationship)
 psychological advice and, 8, 20–22
 sexual, 100–130
 socialization with clients and, 17–18
 spiritual advice and, 22–23
 for students, 157–158
 therapeutic environment and, 7–8
 transference and, 46–58

violation of, 9, 16–23
Professional insecurity, 19–20
Professional roles, 12–13
Professional therapeutic relationship
  (*see* Therapeutic relationship)
Prostitute, being mistaken for, 115–
  119
Psychological counseling, 8, 20–22, 75
 for countertransference, 61–62
 by practitioner, 8, 20–22, 75
 referral for, 75, 93–94
 for sexually abused clients, 108
Psychologically oriented bodywork
  (*see* Emotionally oriented body-
  work)
Public relations, 26–30
Public speaking, 28
Punctuality, 34–35

R
Rape, prevention of, 117–118
Records, medical, privacy of, 38
Referrals
 by clients, 76, 143–144
 for clients, 61, 72, 93–94
 kickbacks and, 144
 rewards for, 143–144
Refunds, 141–142
Refusal
 to accept treatment, 15, 34
 to treat client, 15, 73–74
Reiki, 181
Related readings, 177–178
Relatives, as clients, 150–152
Religious beliefs, 22–23
Reporting, of sexual boundary viola-
  tions, 129
Rescue attitude, 137
Respect
 for clients, 67–68
 for practitioners, 68
Right of refusal
 of client, 15, 34
 of practitioner, 15, 73–74
Role playing, 98
Roles, professional, 12–13
Rolfing, 181
Romantic feelings, 18, 55–56, 59, 61,
  66–67, 101–106 (*see also* Sexual
  boundaries)
Rosen, Marion, 56

Rosen Method, 181
Rubenfeld Synergy Method, 181
Rubin, Paul, 55

S
Safety
  client, 2–3
  practitioner, 117–118
Sales, product, 23, 72–73, 154–155
Schapera, Vivien, 149
Scheduling
  guidelines for, 35–36
  by telephone, 30
Scholl, Bill, 109
Scope of practice, 19, 78, 95
Secrets, 107, 167 (*see also* Confidentiality)
Seductive clients, 125–126 (*see also* Sexual boundaries)
Seductive practitioners, 126–128
Self-presentation, 26–31
Setting limits, 96–98
  financial boundaries and, 134–135
  sexual boundaries and, 119
Sex-seeking clients, 115–123
Sexual assaults, prevention of, 117–118
Sexual boundaries, 18, 61, 66–67, 100–130
  for client, 100–113
  client complaints and, 123–127
  countertransference and, 59, 125–127
  disrobing and, 111
  draping and, 111
  dual relationships and, 106
  erections and, 120–123
  ethical aspects of, 66–70, 73–75, 123–127
  gender dynamics and, 126–127
  intrusive work and, 112
  language and, 111
  locked doors and, 111
  physical affection and, 112
  predatory practitioners and, 127–130
  professional appearance and, 110
  romantic/sexual attraction and, 18, 55–56, 59, 61, 66–67, 101–106
  self-presentation and, 116–117, 119–120

setting limits and, 119
  for sex-seeking clients, 115–123
  for sexually abused clients, 107–110, 112
  transference and, 55–56, 69, 125–127
  unintentional touching and, 112
  violation of, 125–127
Sexual harassment, 127–130
  unfounded accusations of, 124, 128–129
Sexual predators, 127–130
Sexually abused clients, 41–42, 107–110, 112
Sliding-scale fees, 136–139
Socialization, with clients, 17–18, 37, 66–67, 69–70, 103, 148–152 (*see also* Dual relationships)
Somatic practitioners (*see also* Manual therapists), 181
Soundproofing, 38–39
Speaking engagements, 28
Spiritual advice, 22–23
Structural bodywork, framework for, 41
Students, dual relationships and, 157–158
Supervision, 163–164
  benefits of, 163–164, 166–169
  getting started with, 169–170
  group, 165
  versus consultation, 163 (*see also* Consultation)
    definition of, 161
    sharing experiences and, 77
  when to use, 164
Supplements, sale of, 23, 72–73, 154–155
Support groups, peer, 164–166, 170–171

T
Talking
  by client, 20–22
  by therapist, 17–18
Tattoos, 110
Telephone calls, 28–31, 37, 38
  after abrupt termination of therapy, 42
  initial, 30–31
  screening of, 117
  during therapy sessions, 36
Thayer, Brian, 98

Therapeutic contract, 12
Therapeutic environment, 26, 31–33
    (*see also* Work space)
Therapeutic relationship, 7–8, 12–24
  client-centered nature of, 13–14
  client's rights in, 13–15
  confidentiality in, 14 (*see also* Con-
    fidentiality)
  consistency in, 14–15
  control issues in, 86–87
  definition of, 12
  elements of, 12–15
  lawsuits and, 80–83
  money and, 132–133
  power and control in, 86–87
  termination of, 96
  therapist's rights in, 13–15
Therapy sessions
  client expectations for, 34
  communication during, 87–91
  framework guidelines for, 33–40 (*see
    also* Framework(s))
  interruption of, 36
  scheduling of, 30, 35–36
  starting/ending on time, 34–35
Tips, 142–143
Trades
  complications of, 152–154
  dual relationships and, 146–147,
    152–154 (*see also* Dual rela-
    tionships)
  financial boundaries and, 133
  transference and, 106
Trager Approach, 181
Transference, 46–58
  acknowledgment of, 56–58
  captive audience and, 54–55
  client passivity and, 53–54
  communication and, 84
  consultation about, 102–103
  countertransference and, 51–52,
    58–63 (*see also* Countertrans-
    ference)

  dealing with, 56–58, 125–127
  deep emotional work and, 105–106
  definition of, 47
  dependency and, 55
  dual relationships and, 106, 155–156
  in everyday life, 50
  informed consent and, 79
  negative, 48–49
  as normal process, 50
  positive, 48, 55–56, 101–103
  sexual abuse and, 107–110
  sexual boundaries and, 55–56,
    101–103, 125–127
  signs of, 53–56
  socialization with clients and, 148
Traumatized clients, 41–42, 107–110,
  112

U
Undressing, 111

V
Voice mail, 28–30

W
Websites, 28, 117
Weekend workshop syndrome, 19
Wiltsie, Charles, 126
Wooten, Sandra, 34
Work space
  cleanliness of, 32–33
  in-home, 30–32
  location of, 30–32
  personal items in, 32
  preparation of, 32–33
  soundproofing of, 38–39
Workshops
  benefits of, 164–165
  financial, 144–145

Z
Zimmerman, Janet, 55